Ketogenic Diet Cookbook

The Complete Keto Diet Cookbook With Delicious, Effortless, Low Carbs and High-Fat Recipes. Reset Your Metabolism and Start to Eat Healthy Achieving Permanent Weight Loss

By

Ava Spencer

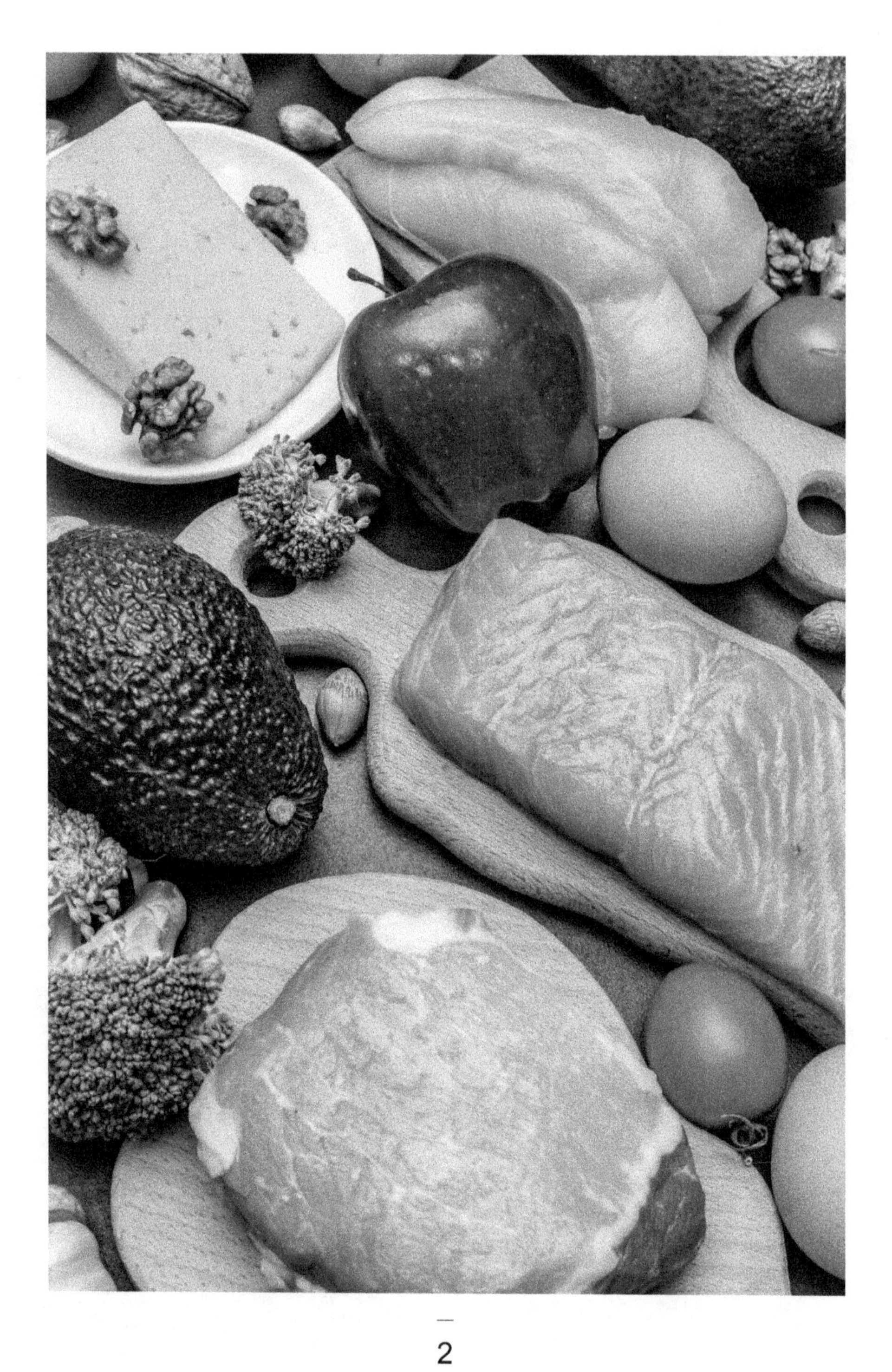

Table of Contents

The information in the following pages is broadly considered a truthful and accurate account of facts and as such, any inattention, use, or misuse of the information in question by the reader will render any resulting actions solely under their purview. There are no scenarios in which the publisher or the original author of this work can be in any fashion deemed liable for any hardship or damages that may befall them after undertaking information described herein.

Additionally, the information in the following pages is intended only for informational purposes and should thus be thought of as universal. As befitting its nature, it is presented without assurance regarding its prolonged validity or interim quality. Trademarks that are mentioned are done without written consent and can in no way be considered an endorsement from the trademark holder.

Introduction

The path to a perfect body and good physical health was very thorny for me. The only one wish which I was making for my birthdays for many years was to be a slim and beautiful girl. Alas, everything can't be as in fairy tales and the miracle didn't happen; my mirror was still showing the same fat, pimple girl. In childhood, the problem of overweight didn't bother me much; I can say that I didn't care about it at all, I didn't know that weight would be momentous for me. I was an ordinary smiling child, playing with my peers, going to school, and traveling with my parents. That time my chubby cheeks seemed very sweet to everyone. But that was then. At 11-year-old, I went to middle school. New people, new teachers, I had no friends at all. Mentally I was broken. I counted the minutes until the end of the last lesson, to quickly sit in my mom's car and leave school. I started to eat a lot. Now I see that in this way I stuck stress, but then the food served as my antidepressant. Dozens of hamburgers, fried potatoes, coke – they were "my best friends". In addition to everything, I started to have horrible skin problems, it seemed to me that there was no place on my face wherever they hadn't appeared yet. Time passed and I no longer loved my reflection in the mirror even in 1%. I couldn't wear the clothes that I liked. I usually wore oversized shorts and t-shirts. I couldn't afford to wear a short dress and high heels. At 15-year-old me was weighted more than 270lbs. I remember what I felt in those days, as it is happening now. I felt anger, irritation, hatred, and self-loathing. That prom party was the most terrible day of my life. Thank God it's over!

In those years, the keto diet was not very popular, fasting and drinking diets (which, as you already know, did not help me much) were more popular. Perhaps I wouldn't do anything, but my health problems were becoming more serious. It seemed that my body was simply screaming: please help me!

I remember the day that changed my life on a dime. I came to the clinic with pain in my stomach. But this time, I not only received painkillers but also found a mentor and friend. This was my physician. She had examined me and recommended to go on a diet. I didn't want to do something and was categorically against it. However, my mind changed when she said: love your body, care about it, and it will thank you. What was my surprise when the diet turned out to be very simple to follow. Is it so easy to love myself? As you could understand I am talking about my favorite keto diet. Every day I was eating a maximum of proteins and a minimum of carbohydrates. That meant to consume meat, poultry, and fish and make restrictions for vegetables, fruits, and sweets. After 2 weeks, I lost 83lbs, and further results were getting better and better. All this time I was under the supervision of a doctor and this yielded results. A year later, I completely changed all the clothes in my wardrobe and oh my God I was able to wear a short dress and skirts! Now I can say that I am the happiest person. It happened because I fall in love with myself and started treated my body as a diamond. My life was filled with bright colors, I have a beloved husband, children, work, friends, I am healthy and like myself in the mirror. I am telling this story a prove that the right diet can solve almost all problems with body and health. It is a fact that our body is capable to deal with dramatic changes, it is only worth loving it. Never rest on your laurels, never give up and forbid people to say that you cannot do something. You are already a great fellow that you bought this cookbook and decided to take a step ahead in the direction to your dream. Let this book become your ray of hope, a lifesaver on the way to your wonderful transformation. If you believe in yourself and love your body, believe me, the result won't be long in coming. You will see in the mirror a completely new version of yourself, updated physically and mentally! Just trust the keto diet and your inner voice. Set a goal today and start the way of achieving it right now. Don't try to do all in one time; let it be small step day by day. Exactly now, this is the right time to start creating a new version of you. If this diet was able to change my life, I'm sure it will help you too!

Ketogenic Recipes for Breakfast

Butter Eggs

Prep time: 10 minutes
Cook time: 15 minutes
Servings: 4

Ingredients:

- 1 teaspoon garlic powder
- 2 tablespoons butter
- 1 teaspoon ground paprika
- 6 eggs, hard-boiled

Method:

1. Peel and cut the eggs into halves.
2. Then melt butter in the skillet and add egg halves and roast them for 1 minute.
3. Sprinkle the eggs with garlic powder and ground paprika.

Nutritional info per serve: Calories 149, Fat 8.6, Fiber 0.3, Carbs 1.3, Protein 8.6

Sausage Sandwich

Prep time: 10 minutes
Cook time: 15 minutes
Servings: 4

Ingredients:

- 4 eggs
- 1 tablespoon butter
- 1 teaspoon ground black pepper
- 8 lettuce leaves
- 4 sausages

Method:

1. Toss the butter in the pan and melt it.
2. Crack the eggs inside and add sausages.
3. Close the lid and cook the ingredients for 5-8 minutes.
4. Then put the eggs and sausages on the lettuce leaves.

Nutritional info per serve: Calories 135, Fat 8.2, Fiber 0.2, Carbs 1, Protein 8.2

Beef Bowl

Prep time: 15 minutes
Cook time: 10 minutes
Servings: 1

Ingredients:

- 4 ounces ground beef
- 1 oz avocado, chopped
- 1 tomato, chopped
- 1 tablespoon butter
- 1 teaspoon chili powder
- 2 oz fresh cilantro, chopped

Method:

1. Put butter in the pan and melt it.
2. Add ground beef and add chili powder and cilantro.
3. Cook the ground beef for 10 minutes on medium heat.
4. Transfer the meat in the bowls and top with tomato and avocado.

Nutritional info per serve: Calories 403, Fat 25, Fiber 5.1, Carbs 8.4, Protein 37.1

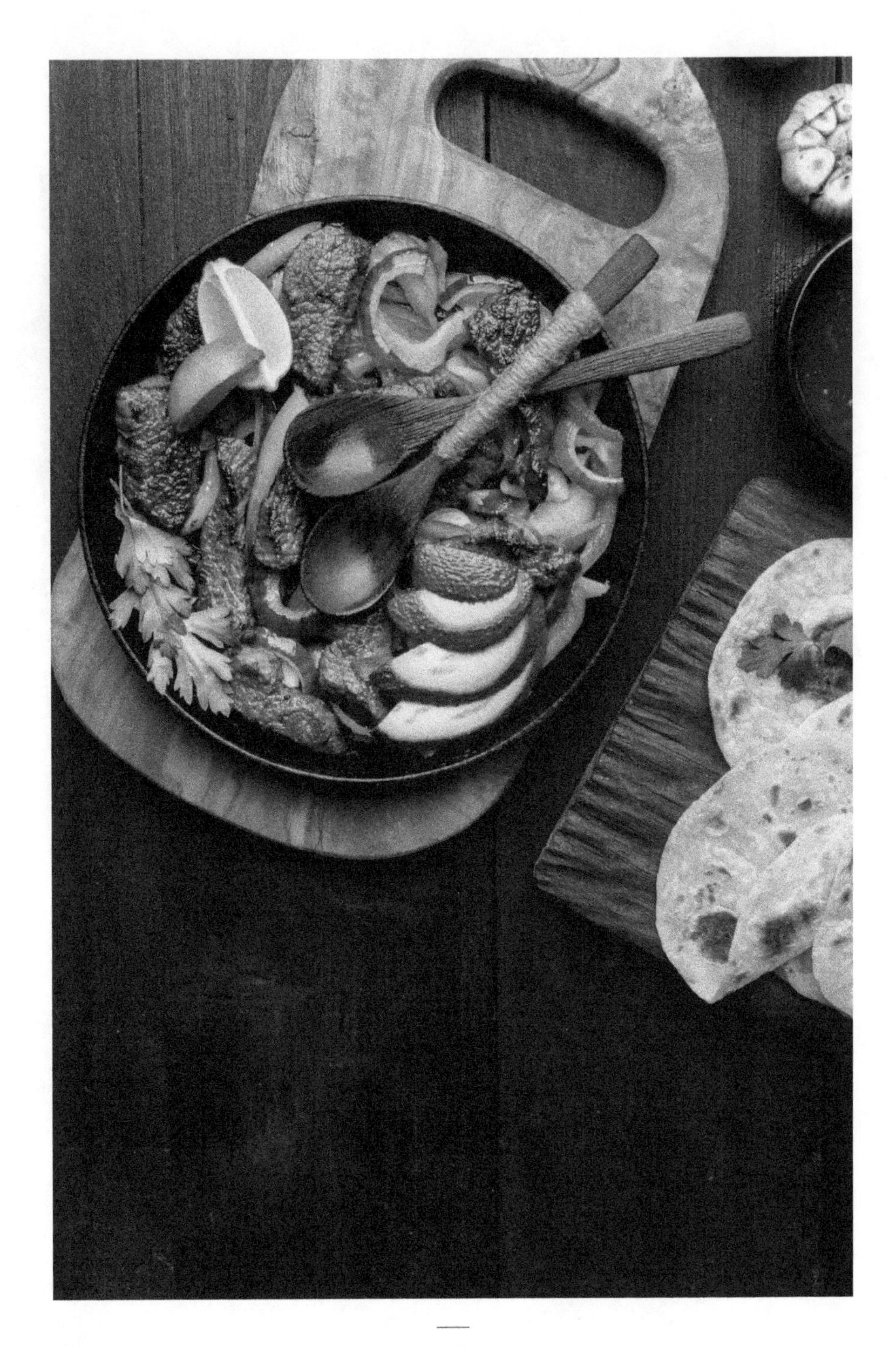

Vanilla Pancakes

Prep time: 10 minutes
Cook time: 10 minutes
Servings: 4

Ingredients:

- 1.5 cups almond flour
- 1 teaspoon vanilla extract
- 3 eggs, beaten
- 1 teaspoon baking powder
- 1 teaspoon Erythritol
- 2 tablespoons avocado oil

Method:

1. Pour avocado oil in the skillet and heat it well.
2. Meanwhile, mix all remaining ingredients in the bowl and whisk until smooth.
3. Pour the small amount of almond flour mixture in the hot skillet and flatten in the shape of the pancake.
4. Roast the pancakes for 1 minute per side on medium-low heat.

Nutritional info per serve: Calories 313, Fat 13.2, Fiber 4.8, Carbs 11.6, Protein 13.2

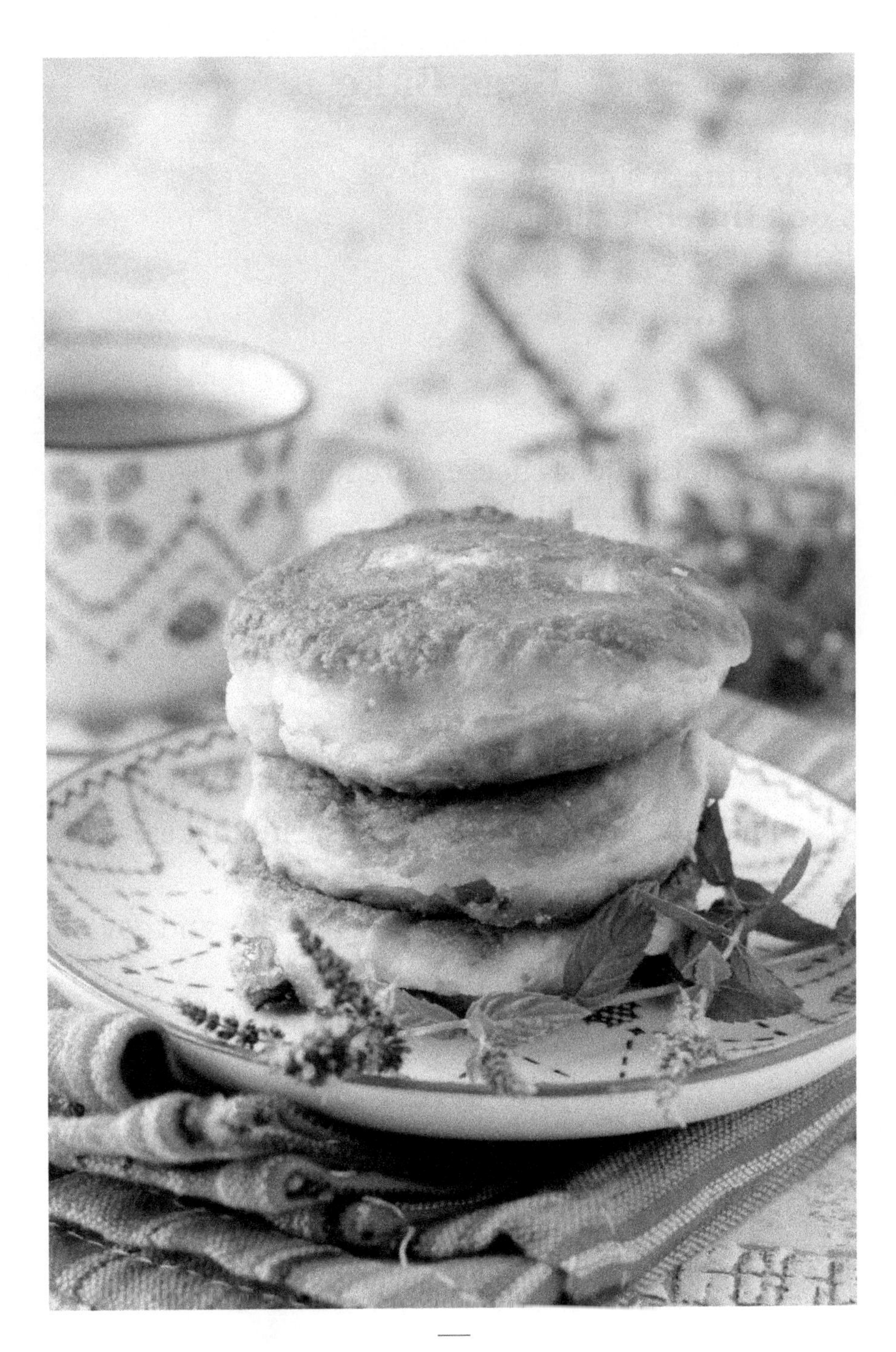

Eggs Bake

Prep time: 10 minutes
Cook time: 15 minutes
Servings: 4

Ingredients:

- 8 eggs, beaten
- 1 cup Cheddar cheese, shredded
- 1 teaspoon chili flakes
- 1 cup spinach, chopped
- 4 teaspoons butter
- ½ teaspoon onion powder

Method:

1. Grease the ramekins with butter.
2. Then mix cheese with eggs, chili flakes, spinach, and onion powder.
3. Pour the mixture in the ramekins and cover with foil.
4. Bake the meal at 365F for 15 minutes.

Nutritional info per serve: Calories 276, Fat 18.4, Fiber 0.2, Carbs 1.6, Protein 18.4

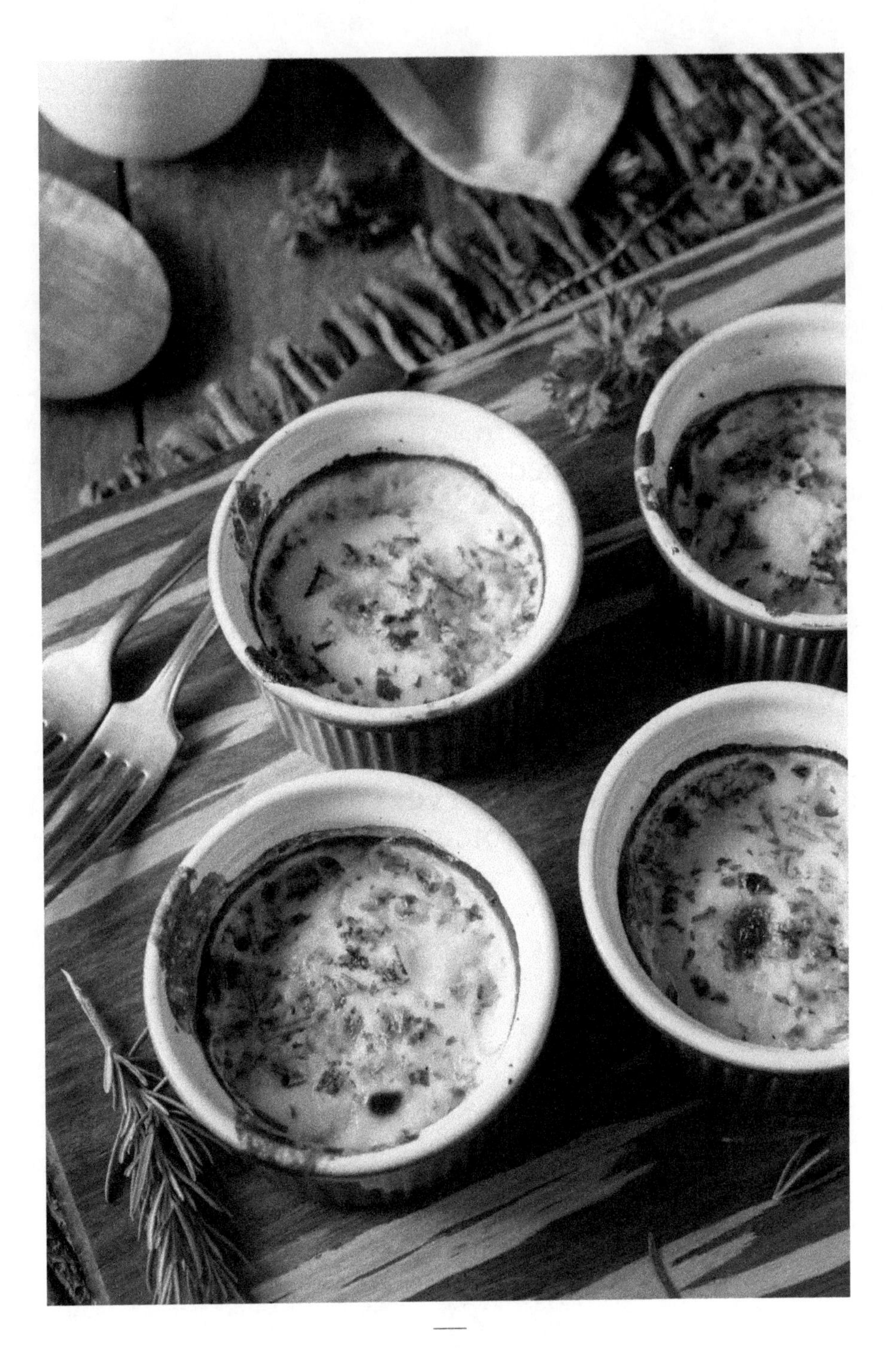

Coconut Smoothie

Prep time: 5 minutes
Servings: 2

Ingredients:

- 1 cup of coconut milk
- 1 cup fresh spinach
- 2 pecans, grinded
- 1 cup fresh parsley

Method:

1. Put all ingredients in the food processor and blend until smooth.
2. Ladle the smoothie in the glasses.

Nutritional info per serve: Calories 388, Fat 5.6, Fiber 5.5, Carbs 11.1, Protein 624

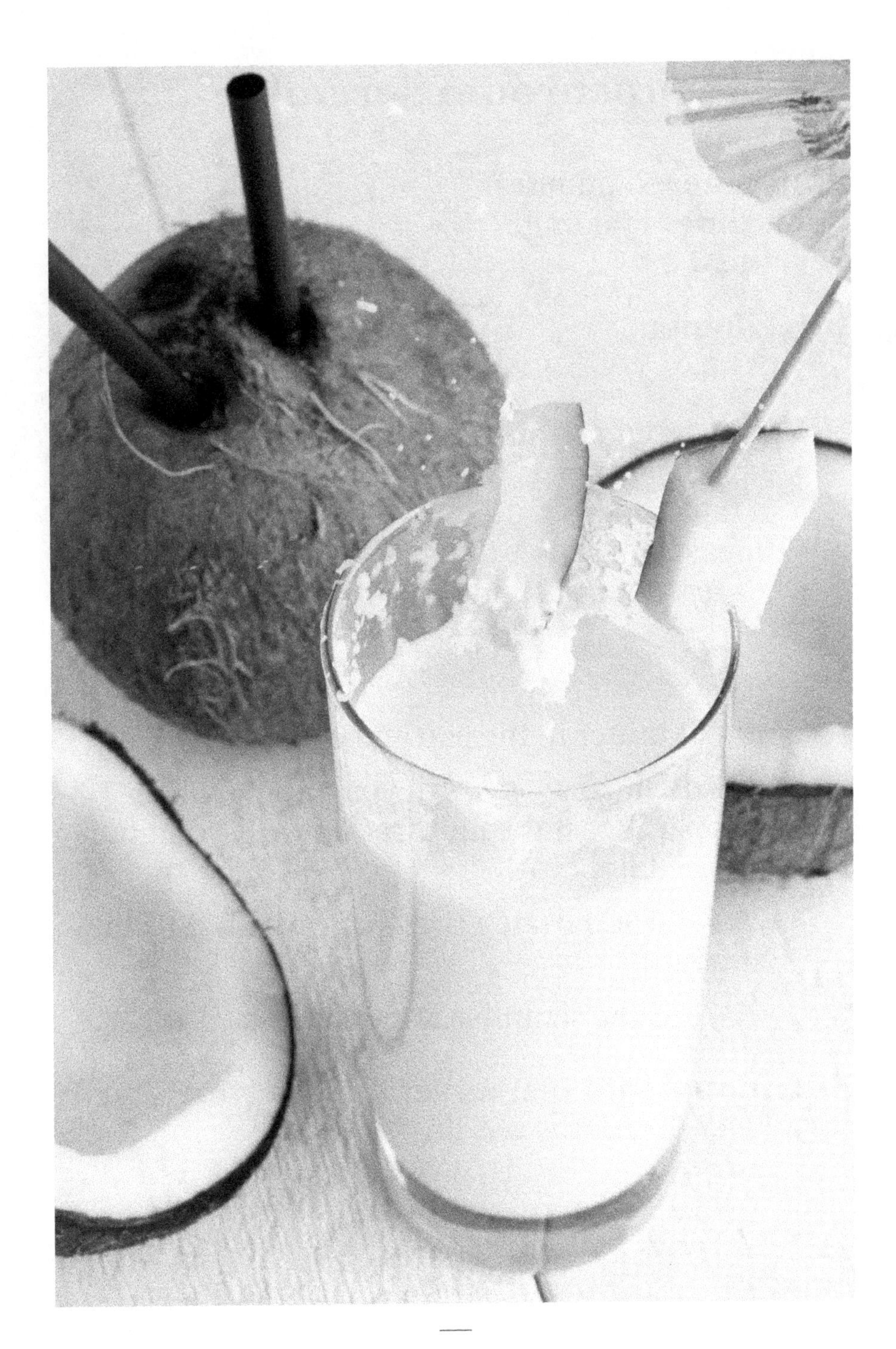

Mushroom Scramble

Prep time: 10 minutes
Cook time: 15 minutes
Servings: 2

Ingredients:

- 1 cup cremini mushrooms, chopped
- 5 eggs, beaten
- 2 tablespoons butter
- 1 teaspoon salt
- ½ teaspoon ground black pepper

Method:

1. Put butter in the pan and melt it.
2. Add mushrooms, salt, and ground black pepper. Roast the mushrooms for 5-10 minutes on medium heat.
3. Then add beaten eggs and carefully stir the mixture.
4. Cook the scramble for 3 minutes.

Nutritional info per serve: Calories 270, Fat 14.9, Fiber 0.4, Carbs 2.7, Protein 14.9

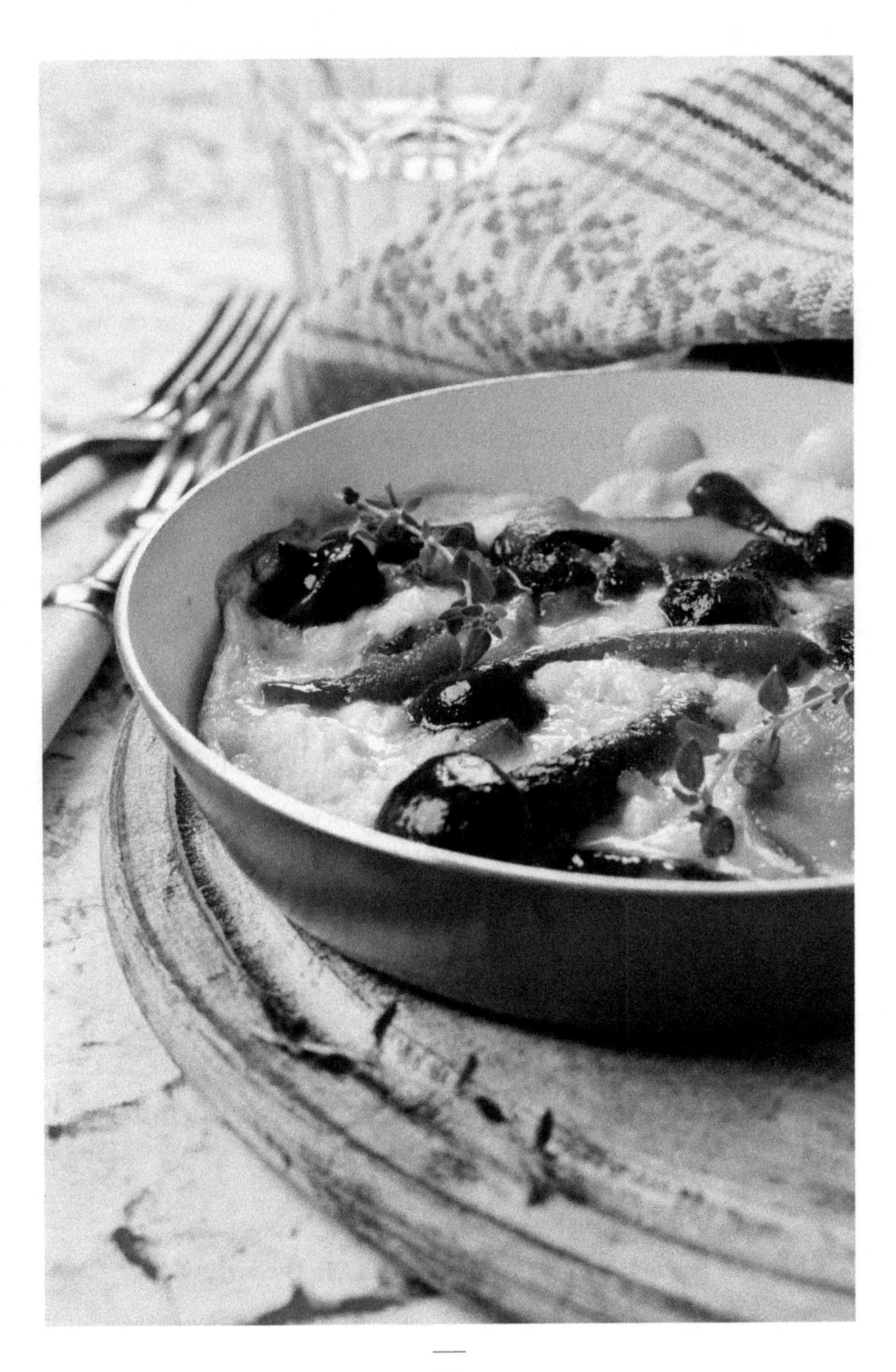

Bacon Muffins

Prep time: 10 minutes
Cook time: 12 minutes
Servings: 4

Ingredients:

- 4 bacon slices, cooked, chopped
- 4 eggs, beaten
- 4 tablespoons almond flour
- 1 teaspoon salt
- 1 teaspoon ground turmeric
- 1 tablespoon avocado oil

Method:

1. Brush the muffin molds with avocado oil.
2. After this, in the mixing bowl, mix eggs with almond flour, salt, ground turmeric, and bacon.
3. Pour the batter in the muffin molds (fill ½ part of every mold) and bake at 365F for 12 minutes.

Nutritional info per serve: Calories 214, Fat 16.1, Fiber 1, Carbs 2.7, Protein 14.2

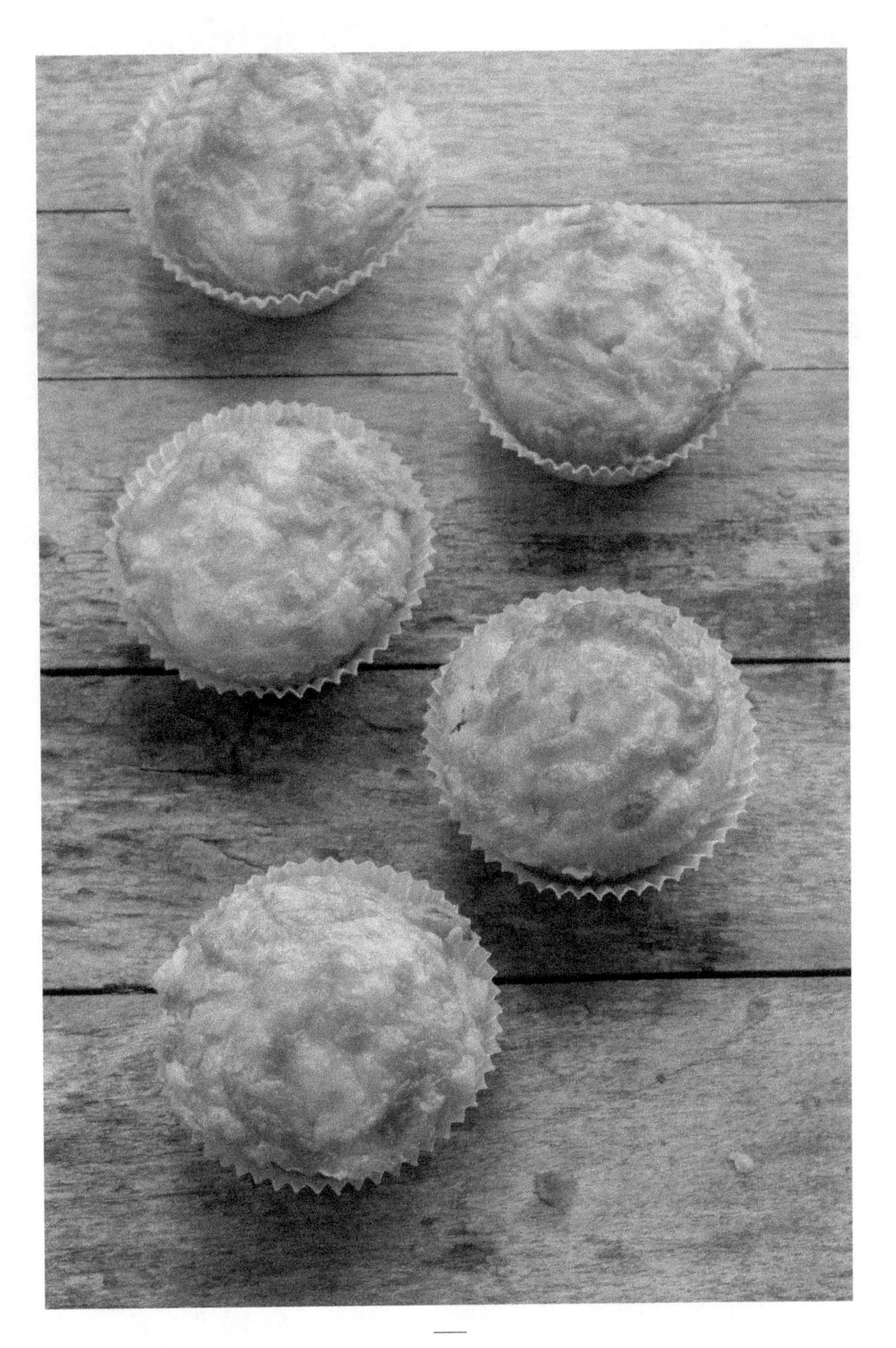

Mozzarella Frittata

Prep time: 10 minutes
Cook time: 25 minutes
Servings: 4

Ingredients:

- 8 eggs, beaten
- ½ teaspoon ground nutmeg
- ½ cup Mozzarella, shredded
- 1 tablespoon coconut cream
- ½ teaspoon ground black pepper
- 1 tablespoon butter

Method:

1. Melt the butter in the skillet.
2. After this, mix eggs with all remaining ingredients.
3. Pour the egg mixture in the hot butter and close the lid.
4. Cook the frittata on low heat with the closed lid for 20 minutes.

Nutritional info per serve: Calories 172, Fat 12.2, Fiber 0.2, Carbs 1.3, Protein 12.2

Eggs in Rings

Prep time: 10 minutes
Cook time: 10 minutes
Servings: 4

Ingredients:

- 1 sweet pepper
- 4 eggs
- 1 teaspoon butter
- ½ teaspoon olive oil
- ¼ teaspoon chili powder

Method:

1. Slice the sweet pepper into 4 rings.
2. Then put butter in the skillet. Add olive oil.
3. After this, add sweet pepper rings and roast them for 1 minute.
4. Flip the pepper rings on another side.
5. Crack the eggs inside pepper rings and sprinkle with chili powder.
6. Cook the eggs for 4 minutes on medium heat.

Nutritional info per serve: Calories 86, Fat 6, Fiber 0.5, Carbs 2.7, Protein 5.9

Ketogenic Recipes for Lunch

Avocado and Chicken Salad

Prep time: 10 minutes
Cook time: 0 minutes
Servings: 2

Ingredients:

- 1 avocado, pitted, peeled, and sliced
- 1 teaspoon chili powder
- 1 tablespoon cream cheese
- 1 chicken breast, grilled and shredded

Method:

1. In the salad bowl mix all ingredients.
2. Shake the salad before serving.

Nutritional info per serve: Calories 347, Fat 23.1, Fiber 7.2, Carbs 9.5, Protein 28.5

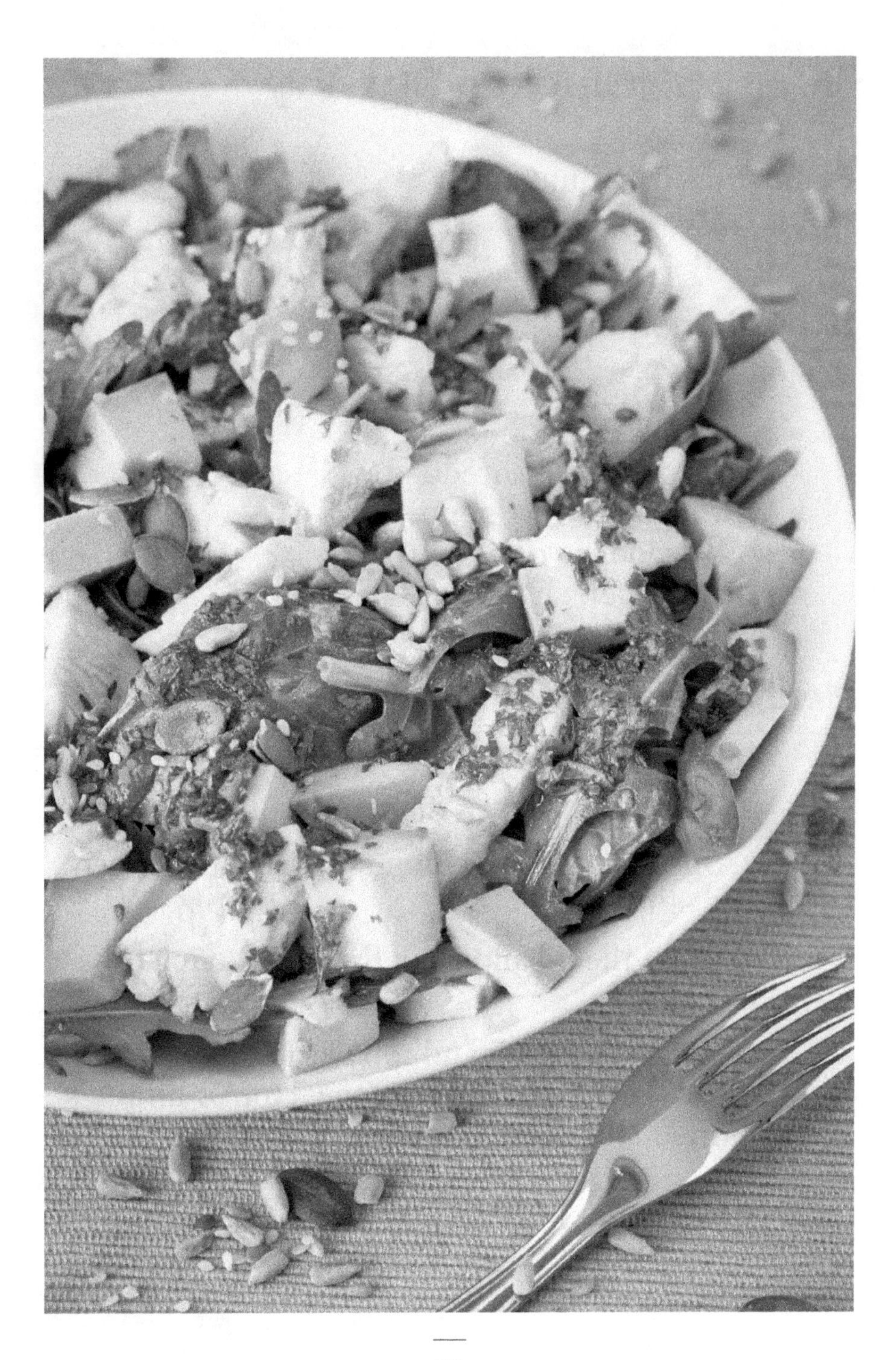

Chicken Stir-Fry

Prep time: 10 minutes
Cook time: 25 minutes
Servings: 4

Ingredients:

- 1-pound chicken fillet, sliced
- 3 oz Mozzarella, shredded
- ½ teaspoon white pepper
- 1 tablespoon avocado oil
- 1 bell pepper, sliced

Method:

1. Pour avocado oil in the skillet and heat well.
2. Then add chicken fillet and bell pepper.
3. Sprinkle the ingredients with white pepper and stir well.
4. Close the lid and cook the mixture for 10 minutes.
5. Then stir it well and top with Mozzarella. Close the lid and cook the meal for 10 minutes more on low heat.

Nutritional info per serve: Calories 290, Fat 12.7, Fiber 0.6, Carbs 3.4, Protein 39.2

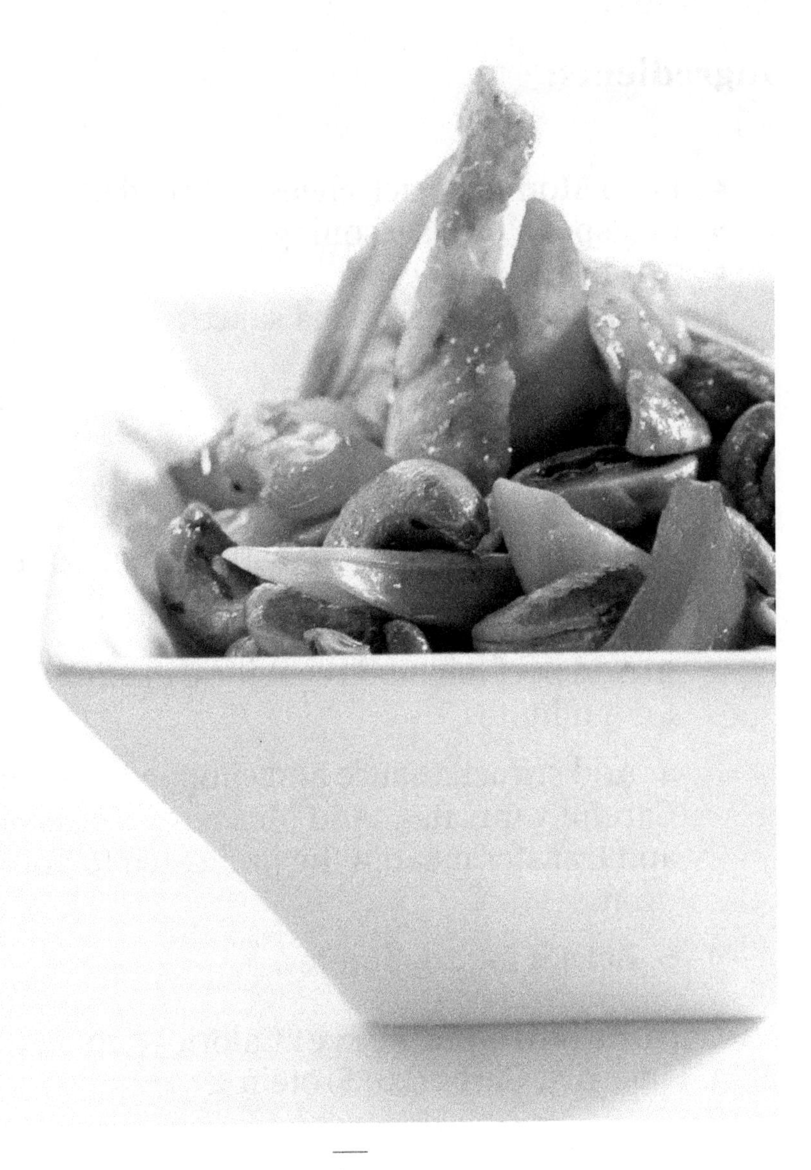

Beef Tacos

Prep time: 10 minutes
Cook time: 25 minutes
Servings: 3

Ingredients:

- 1 cup Monterey jack cheese, shredded
- 1 teaspoon taco seasoning
- 7 oz beef loin, sliced
- 2 teaspoons keto riracha sauce
- 1 tomato, chopped
- 2 tablespoons coconut oil

Method:

1. Sprinkle the beef loin with taco seasonings.

2. Then melt the coconut oil in the pan.

3. Add beef loin and roast it on medium heat for 5 minutes.

4. Add sriracha sauce and chopped tomato. Carefully mix it. 5. Add Monterey jack cheese and transfer meat in the preheated to 360F oven.

6. Bake it for 20 minutes.

Nutritional info per serve: Calories 372, Fat 28.3, Fiber 0.3, Carbs 2.6, Protein 27.1

Salmon Bowl

Prep time: 10 minutes
Cook time: 10 minutes
Servings: 5

Ingredients:

- 12 oz salmon fillet
- ½ teaspoon ground nutmeg
- 1 tablespoon lime juice
- 1 tablespoon canola oil
- 2 cup fresh spinach, chopped
- ½ cup tomatoes, chopped
- 1 teaspoon sesame oil

Method:

1. Heat the sesame oil in the skillet.
2. Then chop the salmon fillet roughly and sprinkle with ground nutmeg.
3. Put it in the hot oil and roast for 2 minutes per side.
4. Then put the fish in the bowl.
5. Add lime juice, canola oil, tomatoes, and fresh spinach.
6. Shake the ingredients gently.

Nutritional info per serve: Calories 130, Fat 8.1, Fiber 0.5, Carbs 1.3, Protein 13.7

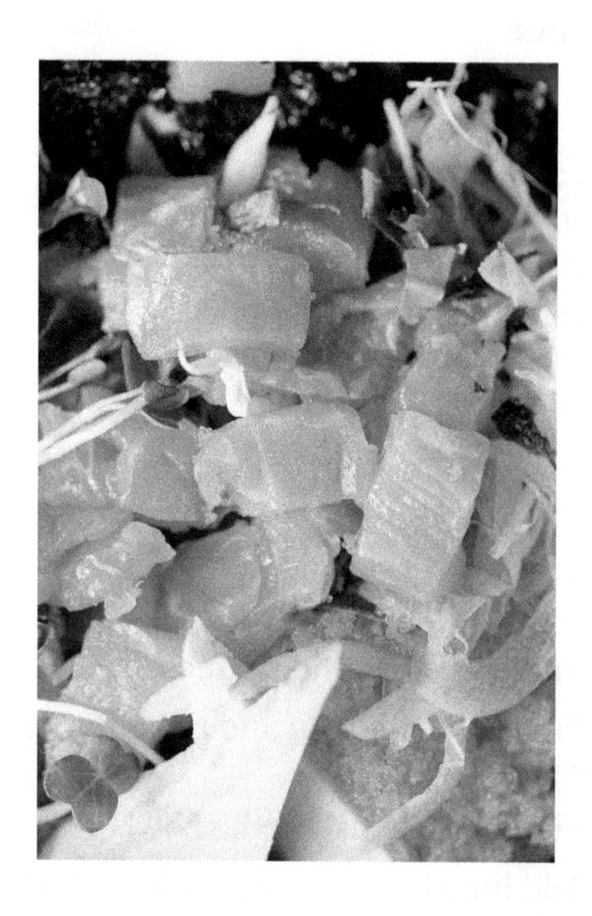

Cauliflower Pizza

Prep time: 15 minutes
Cook time: 10 minutes
Servings: 4

Ingredients:

- 1 tablespoon avocado oil
- 2 tablespoons coconut oil
- 2 cups Cheddar cheese, shredded
- ¼ cup mascarpone cheese
- 1⅓ cup cauliflower florets, steamed

Method:

1. Line the baking tray with cooking paper.
2. Then mash the cauliflower and mix it with avocado oil, coconut oil, and mascarpone.
3. Transfer the mixture in the baking tray and flatten in the shape of the pizza.
4. Top it with cheddar cheese and bake at 360F for 10 minutes.

Nutritional info per serve: Calories 341, Fat 28.1, Fiber 2.4, Carbs 6.3, Protein 17.7

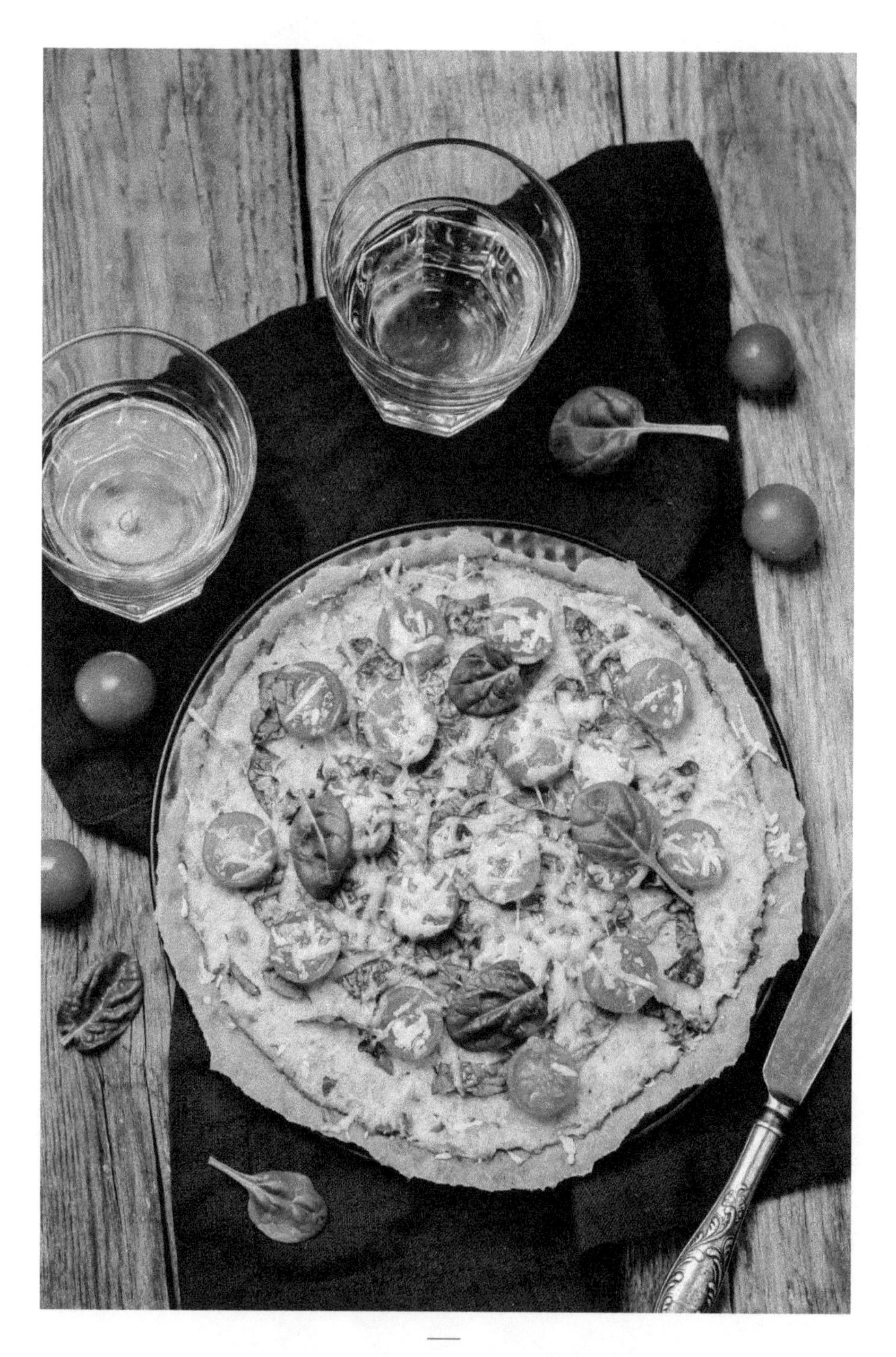

Broccoli and Bacon Bowls

Prep time: 15 minutes
Cook time: 7 minutes
Servings: 4

Ingredients:

- 1 cup broccoli florets
- 1 spring onion, sliced
- 5 oz bacon, fried, chopped
- 5 oz Monterey Jack cheese, grated
- 1 tablespoon ricotta cheese
- 1 tablespoon fresh parsley, chopped
- ½ teaspoon chili powder
- 1 cup water, for cooking

Method:

1. Pour water in the pan and bring it to boil.
2. Add broccoli florets and boil them for 7 minutes.
3. After this, remove broccoli from the water and transfer it in the big bowl.
4. In the separated bowl, mix fresh parsley, chili powder, and ricotta cheese.
5. Melt the mixture and add in the broccoli.
6. Then add Monterey Jack cheese, spring onion, and bacon.

7. Shake the meal well and transfer in the serving bowls.

Nutritional info per serve: Calories 344, Fat 26, Fiber 1, Carbs 4, Protein 23.1

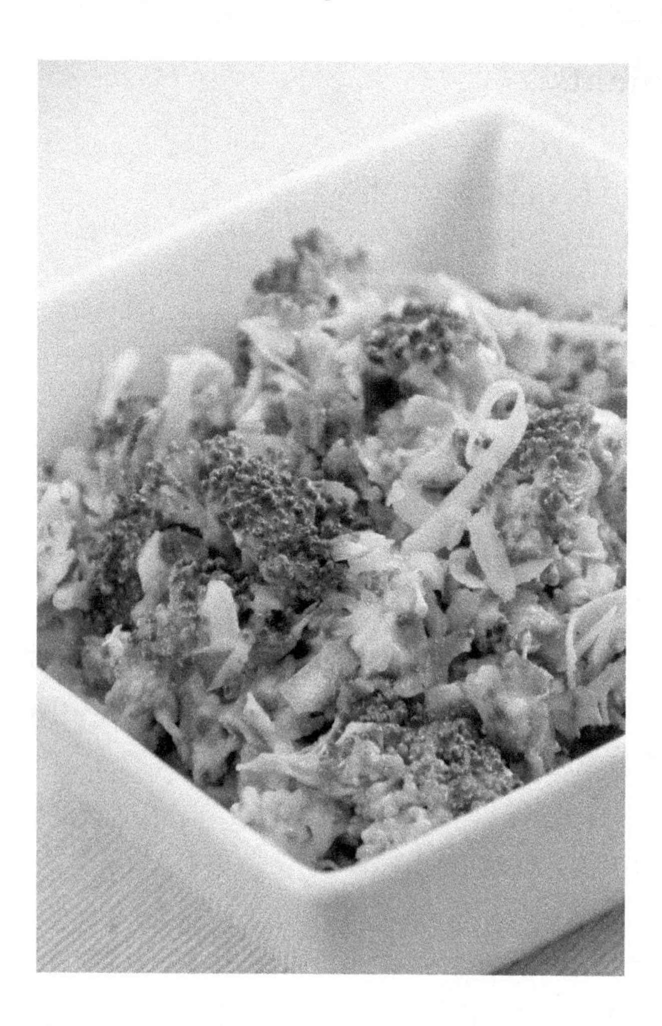

Tomato Pan

Prep time: 10 minutes
Cook time: 25 minutes
Servings: 6

Ingredients:

- ¼ cup bell pepper, chopped
- 2 cups Cheddar cheese, shredded
- 1 teaspoon taco seasoning
- 2 scallions, diced
- 1 tomato, chopped
- ½ cup ground sausages
- 1 tablespoon coconut oil

Method:

1. Melt the coconut oil in the pan and add bell pepper.
2. Roast it for 2 minutes and stir well.
3. Then add scallions and ground sausages.
4. Roast the ingredients for 10 minutes on medium heat.
5. Add all remaining ingredients except Cheddar cheese and roast the meal for 10 minutes.
6. Top the meal with Cheddar cheese.

Nutritional info per serve: Calories 188, Fat 14.8, Fiber 0.6, Carbs 3.3, Protein 10.6

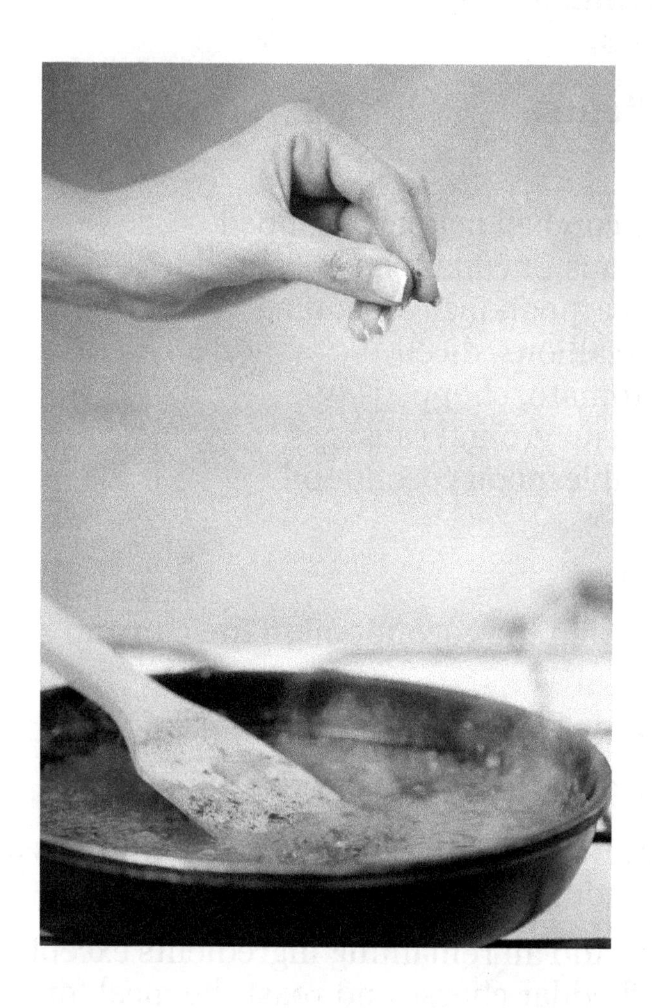

Chicken Tortillas

Prep time: 10 minutes
Cook time: 20 minutes
Servings: 6

Ingredients:

- 1-pound chicken fillet, boiled, chopped
- 1 teaspoon ground black pepper
- ¾ cup coconut cream
- ½ teaspoon chili powder
- 1 teaspoon coconut oil
- 6 keto tortillas

Method:

1. Melt the coconut oil in the pan.
2. Then mix chopped chicken fillet with ground black pepper and chili powder.
3. Transfer the chicken in the melted coconut oil and roast for 5 minutes.
4. Then add coconut cream and cook the chicken for 10 minutes on medium heat.
5. Fill the tortillas with chicken and roll.

Nutritional info per serve: Calories 371, Fat 21.6, Fiber 4.8, Carbs 10, Protein 34.6

Cheddar Pizza

Prep time: 10 minutes
Cook time: 25 minutes
Servings: 6

Ingredients:

- 1½ cups cheddar cheese, shredded
- 1-pound ground beef, cooked
- 1 tomato, chopped
- 1 teaspoon avocado oil
- 1 teaspoon dried basil

Method:

1. Line the baking tray with baking paper.
2. Then mix dried basil with ground beef.
3. Sprinkle the tray with avocado oil and put the ground beef inside.
4. Flatten it in the shape of the pizza and bake at 360F for 15 minutes.
5. Then top the pizza with chopped tomato and cheese.
6. Cook it for 10 minutes more.

Nutritional info per serve: Calories 561, Fat 39.2, Fiber 0.2, Carbs 1.8, Protein 48.8

Halloumi Salad

Prep time: 10 minutes
Cook time: 3 minutes
Servings: 4

Ingredients:

- 4 oz Halloumi cheese
- 8 oz chicken breast, boiled, chopped
- 1 cup lettuce, chopped
- 1 pecan, chopped
- 2 tablespoons avocado oil
- 1 tablespoon lime juice

Method:

1. Preheat the grill to 400F.
2. Slice the halloumi cheese roughly and sprinkle with avocado oil.
3. Grill the cheese for 1 minute per side and put it in the salad bowl.
4. Add chopped chicken and all remaining ingredients.
5. Shake the salad.

Nutritional info per serve: Calories 203, Fat 13.3, Fiber 0.8, Carbs 2, Protein 18.7

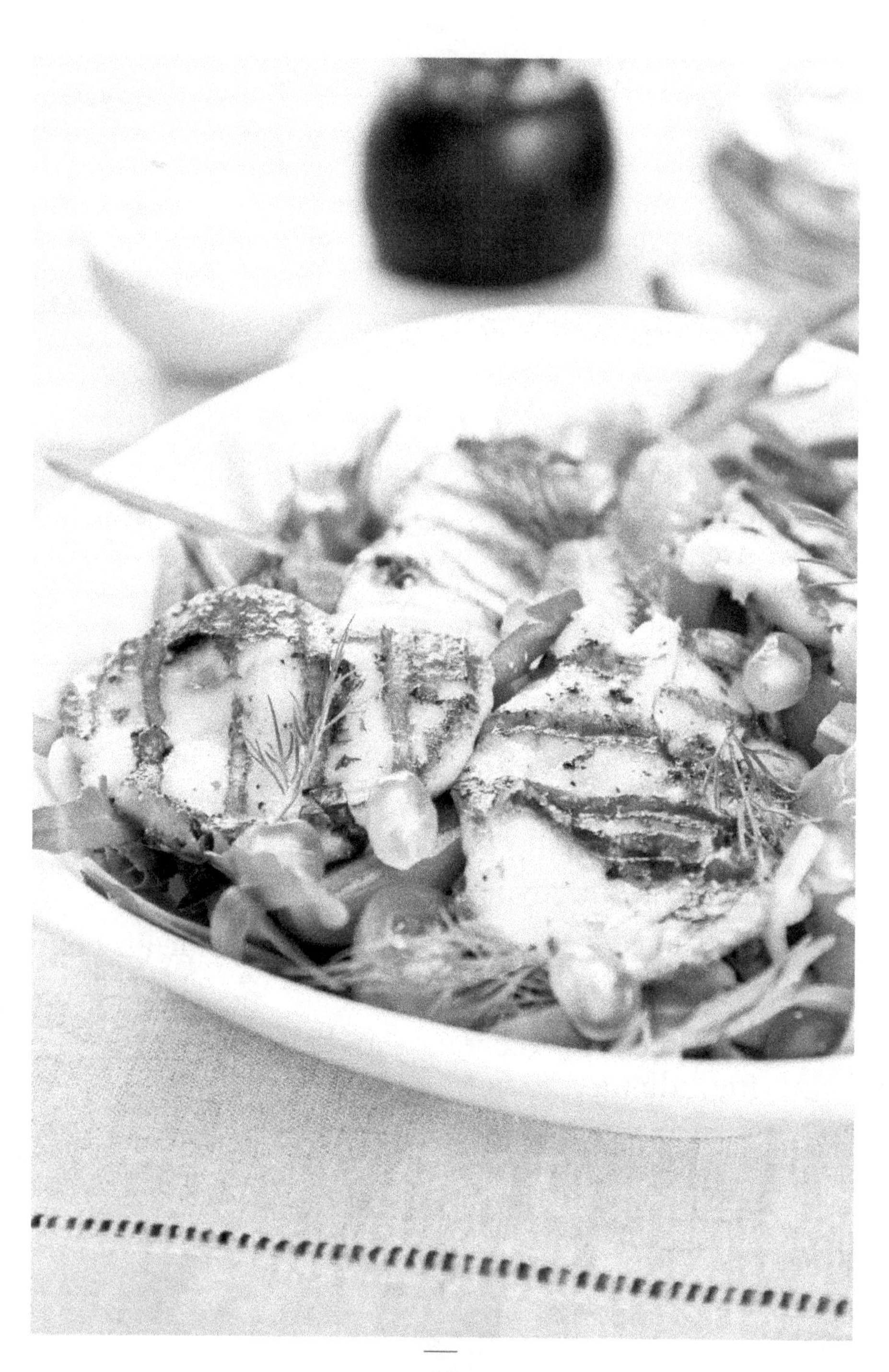

Ketogenic Side Dish Recipes

Cabbage Mix

Prep time: 10 minutes

Cook time: 0 minutes

Servings: 6

Ingredients:

- 2 pounds white cabbage, shredded
- ½ cup turnip, chopped
- 2 tablespoons scallions, chopped
- 2 tablespoons chili powder
- 1 teaspoon garlic powder
- 1 teaspoon ginger powder

Method:

1. In the mixing bowl, mix white cabbage with turnip, scallions, and chili powder.
2. Add garlic powder and ginger powder.
3. Carefully mix the meal and leave for 10 minutes before serving.

Nutritional info per serve: Calories 52, Fat 0.6, Fiber 5, Carbs 11.5, Protein 2.5

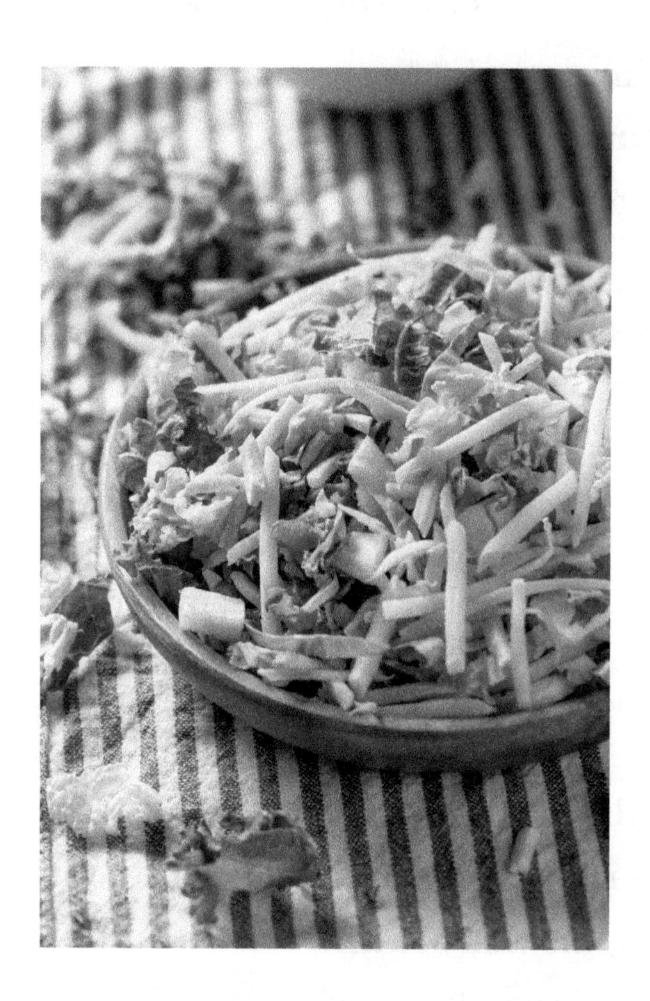

Italian Style Mushrooms

Prep time: 10 minutes

Cook time: 30 minutes

Servings: 4

Ingredients:

- 2 cups cremini mushrooms
- 1 teaspoon Italian seasoning
- 2 tablespoons coconut oil
- ¼ cup coconut cream

Method:

1. Melt the coconut oil in the saucepan.
2. Add mushrooms and roast them for 10 minutes.
3. Then sprinkle them with Italian seasonings and coconut cream.
4. Bake the mushrooms at 360F for 15 minutes.

Nutritional info per serve: Calories 106, Fat 10.8, Fiber 0.6, Carbs 2.4, Protein 1.2

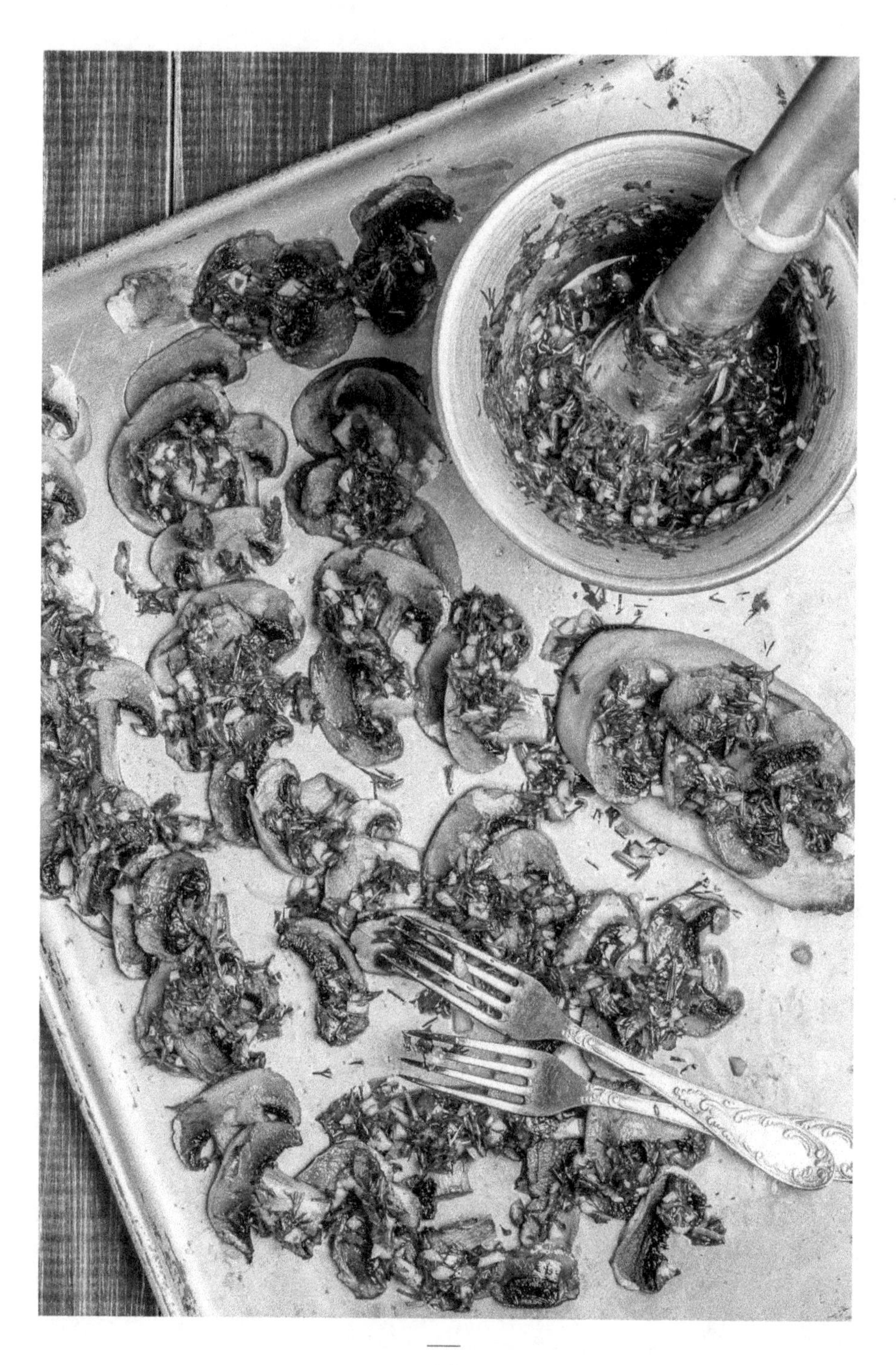

Cheddar Green Beans

Prep time: 10 minutes

Cook time: 20 minutes

Servings: 4

Ingredients:

- ½ cup Cheddar cheese, shredded
- 2 cups green beans, chopped
- 1 teaspoon ground black pepper
- 1 tablespoon olive oil

Method:

1. Sprinkle the green beans with ground black pepper and olive oil and put in the hot skillet.
2. Roast the green beans for 10 minutes on medium heat.
3. Stir them from time to time to avoid burning.
4. Then top the vegetables with cheese and close the lid.
5. Cook the meal on low heat for 10 minutes.

Nutritional info per serve: Calories 105, Fat 8.3, Fiber 2, Carbs 4.4, Protein 4.6

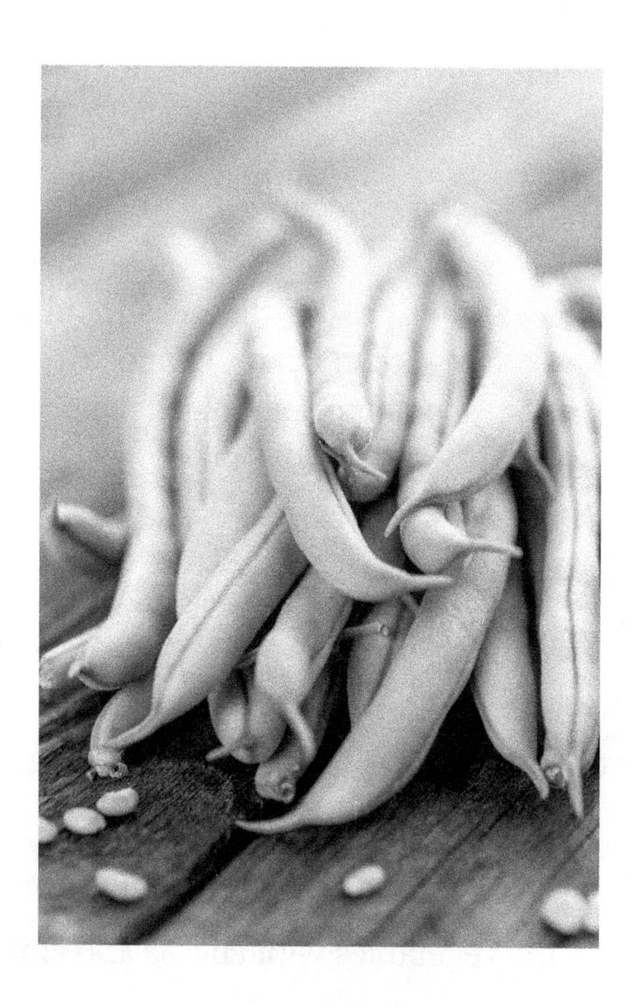

Butter Asparagus

Prep time: 10 minutes

Cook time: 25 minutes

Servings: 4

Ingredients:

- 1.5-pound asparagus
- 2 tablespoons lemon juice
- 1 teaspoon lemon zest, grated
- 4 tablespoons butter
- ¼ cup coconut cream
- ¼ teaspoon chili flakes

Method:

1. Chop the asparagus and put it in the baking tray.
2. Sprinkle the vegetables with lemon juice, lemon zest, butter, coconut cream, and chili flakes.
3. Shake the ingredients and bake at 360F for 25 minutes.

Nutritional info per serve: Calories 173, Fat 15.4, Fiber 4, Carbs 7.7, Protein 4.3

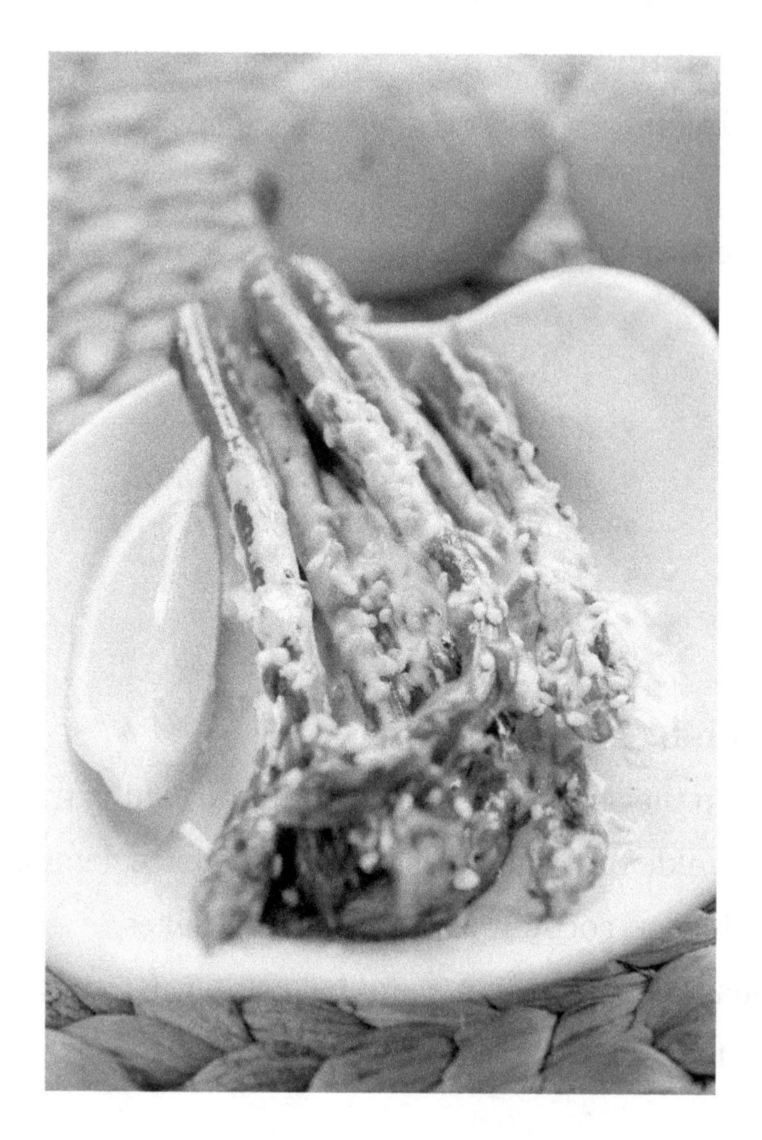

Cauliflower Puree

Prep time: 10 minutes

Cook time: 15 minutes

Servings: 2

Ingredients:

- ¼ cup coconut cream
- 1 cup cauliflower chopped
- 1 teaspoon salt
- 2 cups of water

Method:

1. Pour water in the saucepan.
2. Add cauliflower and boil it for 15 minutes.
3. Then drain water and mash the cauliflower with the help of potato masher.
4. Add all remaining ingredients and carefully mix the meal.

Nutritional info per serve: Calories 82, Fat 7.2, Fiber 1.9, Carbs 4.3, Protein 1.7

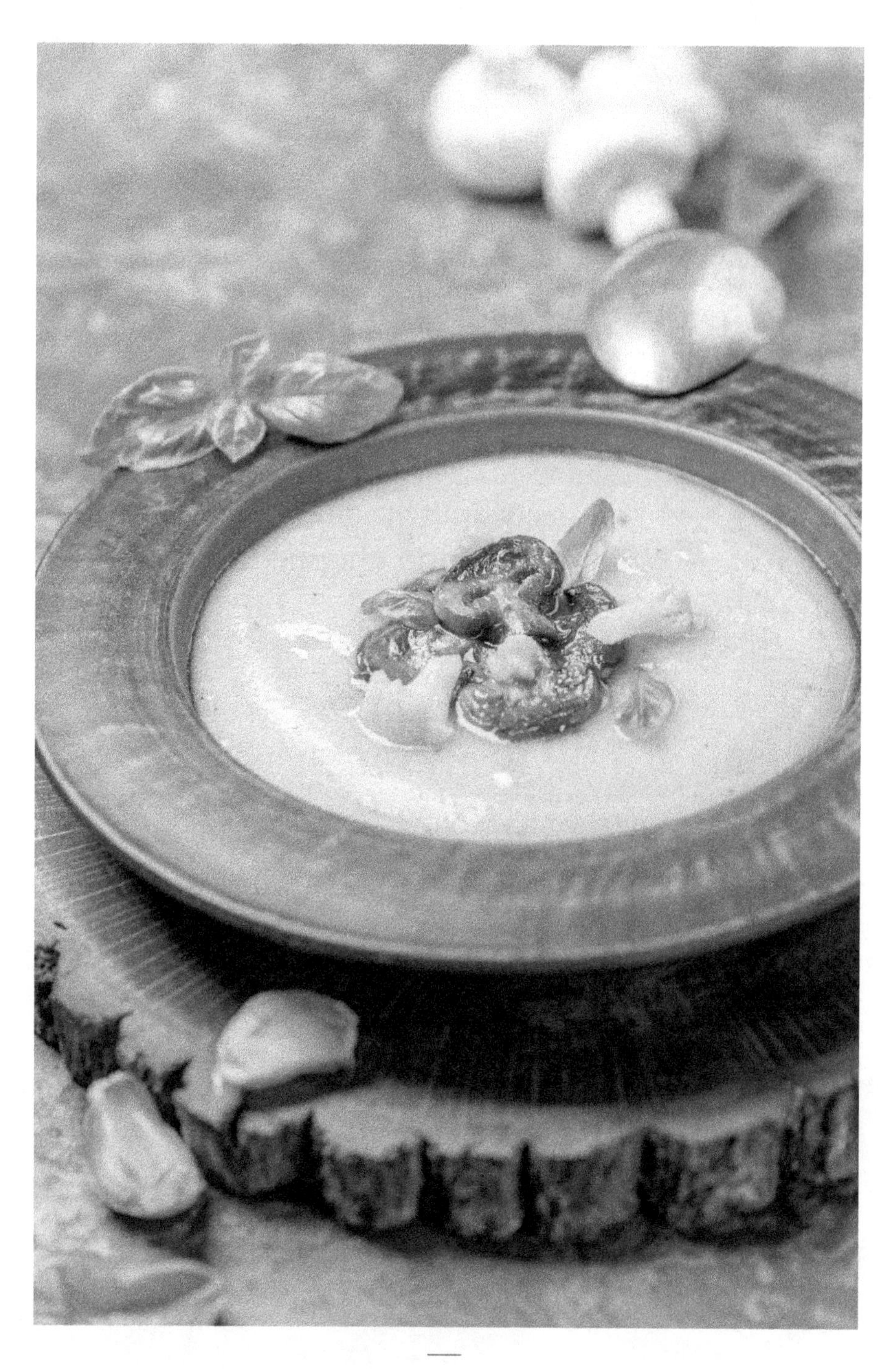

Sesame Brussel Sprouts

Prep time: 10 minutes

Cook time: 6 minutes

Servings: 4

Ingredients:

- 3 cups Brussel sprouts
- 1 teaspoon garlic, minced
- 1 teaspoon sesame seeds
- 1 tablespoon coconut oil
- ½ cup of water

Method:

1. Bring the water to boil.
2. Add Brussel sprouts and boil them for 1 minute.
3. Then transfer them in the hot skillet.
4. Add garlic, sesame seeds, and coconut oil.
5. Carefully mix and cook the meal for 5 minutes on medium heat. Stir it from time to time.

Nutritional info per serve: Calories 63, Fat 4, Fiber 2.6, Carbs 6.4, Protein 2.4

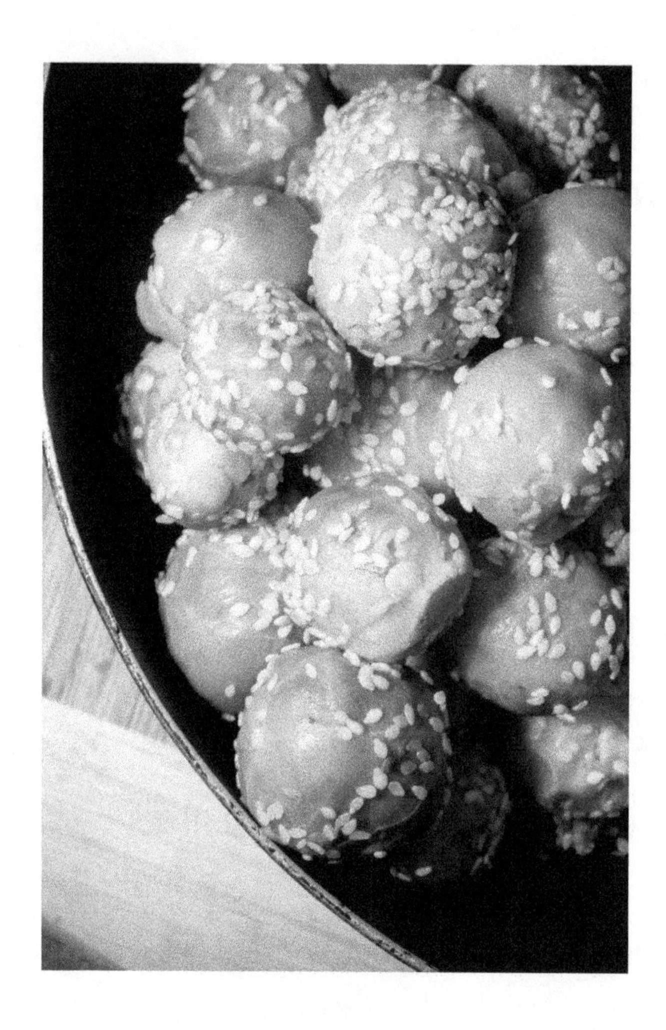

Tarragon Mushrooms

Prep time: 10 minutes

Cook time: 15 minutes

Servings: 4

Ingredients:

- 10 oz cremini mushrooms, sliced
- 2 tablespoons avocado oil
- ½ teaspoon tarragon, dried
- 2 tablespoons apple cider vinegar

Method:

1. Sprinkle the baking tray with avocado oil.

2. Then mix mushrooms with tarragon and apple cider vinegar. 3. Put them in the baking tray and flatten in the layer.

4. Bake the mushrooms at 360F for 15 minutes. Stir them from time to time to avoid burning.

Nutritional info per serve: Calories 30, Fat 1, Fiber 0.8, Carbs 3.4, Protein 1.9

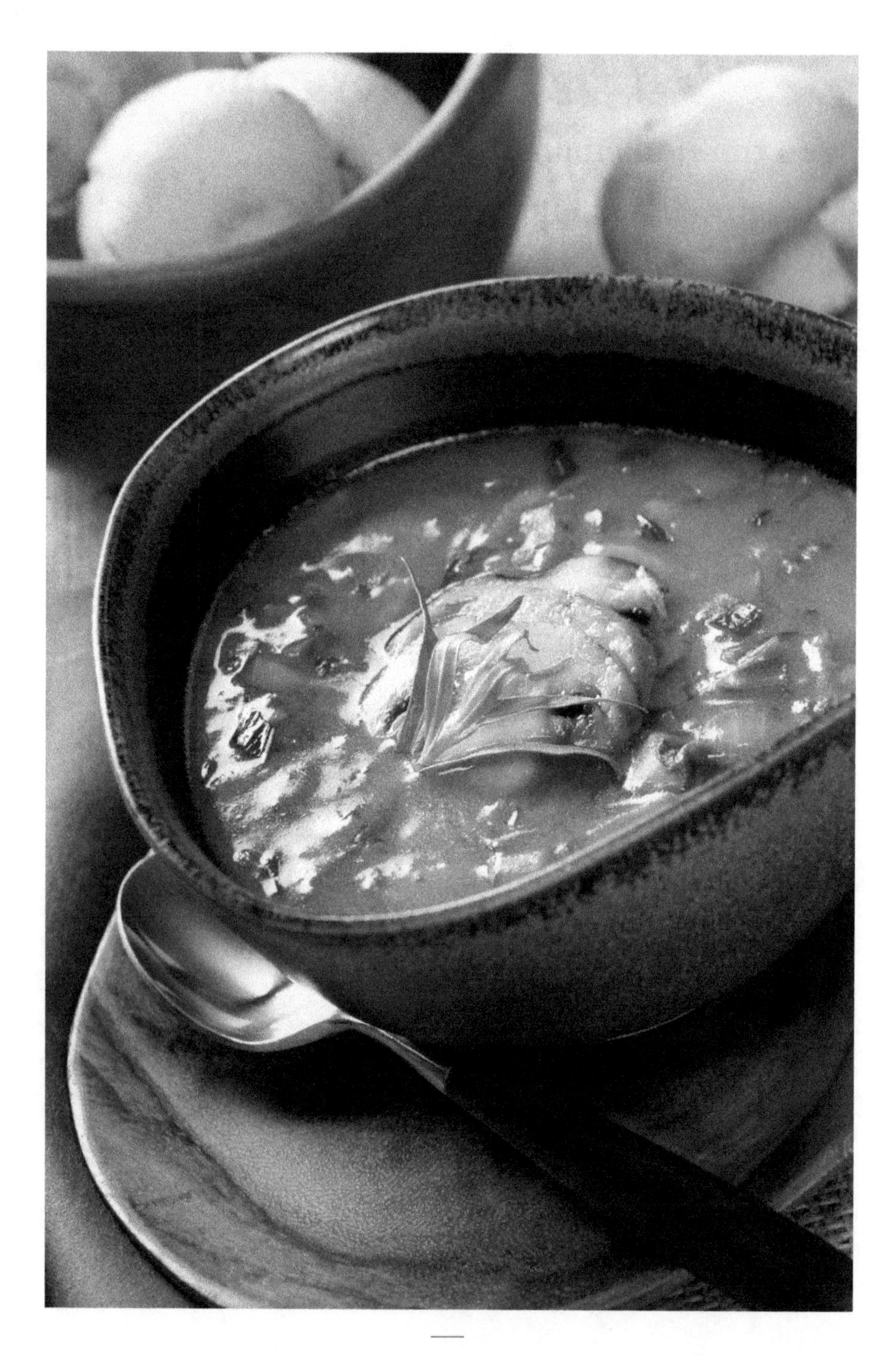

Spinach Mash

Prep time: 5 minutes

Cook time: 5 minutes

Servings: 3

Ingredients:

- 3 cups fresh spinach, chopped
- 1 tablespoon ricotta cheese
- ¼ cup coconut cream
- 1 spring onion, diced
- 1 teaspoon coconut oil
- 1 oz Parmesan, grated

Method:

1. Melt the coconut oil in the saucepan.
2. Add chopped spinach and roast it for 3 minutes on medium heat. 3. Carefully mix the spinach and add ricotta cheese, coconut cream, spring onion, and Parmesan.
4. Carefully mix the spinach until the cheese is melted and remove it from the heat.

Nutritional info per serve: Calories 104, Fat 8.8, Fiber 1.1, Carbs 2.9, Protein 5

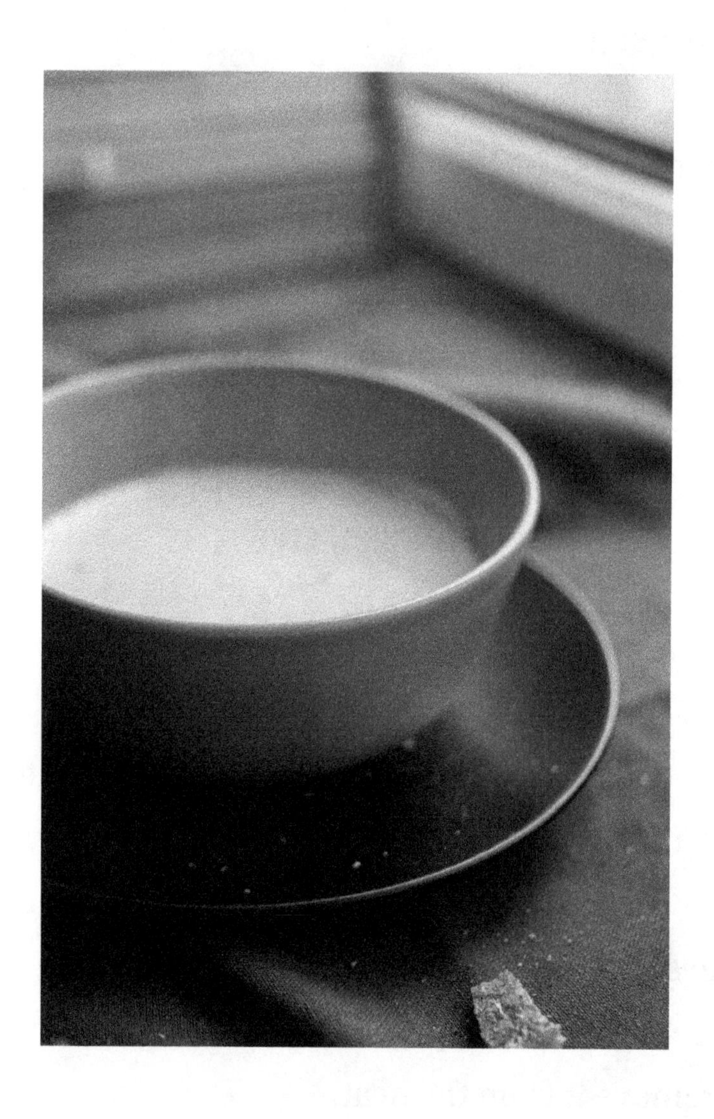

Pepper Brussels Sprouts

Prep time: 10 minutes

Cook time: 11 minutes

Servings: 4

Ingredients:

- 1-pound Brussels sprouts, trimmed and halved
- 1 teaspoon chili powder
- 1 teaspoon garlic powder
- 1 teaspoon avocado oil
- 1 tablespoon apple cider vinegar
- 1 cup of water

Method:

1. Put the Brussel sprouts in the pan and add water. Boil the vegetables for 10 minutes.
2. Then drain water and add all remaining ingredients.
3. Carefully mix the mixture and cook it on medium heat for 1 minute more.

Nutritional info per serve: Calories 56, Fat 0.7, Fiber 4.6, Carbs 11.3, Protein 4.1

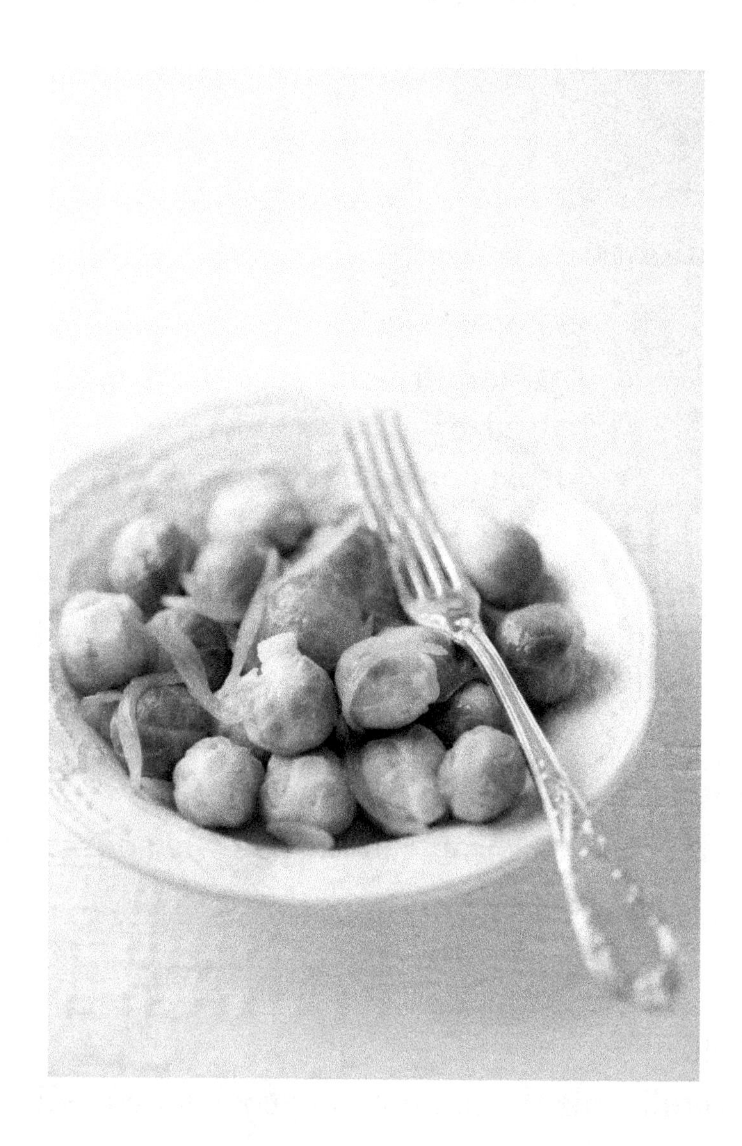

Chili Bok Choy

Prep time: 10 minutes

Cook time: 7 minutes

Servings: 4

Ingredients:

- 1-pound bok choy
- 1 teaspoon chili flakes
- 2 tablespoons avocado oil
- 1 teaspoon lemon juice

Method:

1. Preheat the avocado oil in the skillet.
2. Slice the bok choy and put it in the hot oil.
3. Sprinkle it with lemon juice and chili flakes and roast for 2 minutes per side.

Nutritional info per serve: Calories 24, Fat 1.1, Fiber 1.5, Carbs 2.9, Protein 1.8

Spinach Sauce

Prep time: 10 minutes

Cook time: 10 minutes

Servings: 4

Ingredients:

- 1 tablespoon coconut oil
- 2 cups fresh spinach, chopped
- 1 pecan, chopped
- 2 oz Provolone, grated
- 1 teaspoon minced garlic

Method:

1. Melt the coconut oil and put spinach in it.

2. Add pecan, cheese, and minced garlic.

3. Carefully mix the mixture and cook it for 5 minutes.

4. Then blend it with the help of the immersion blender until smooth.

Nutritional info per serve: Calories 108, Fat 9.7, Fiber 0.7, Carbs 1.6, Protein 4.5

Ketogenic Meat Recipes

Lemon Pork Belly

Prep time: 10 minutes

Cook time: 30 minutes

Servings: 6

Ingredients:

- 1-pound pork belly
- 2 cups of water
- 1 teaspoon dried thyme
- 1 teaspoon salt
- 1 teaspoon peppercorn
- 2 tablespoons lemon juice

Method:

1. Bring the water to boil and add peppercorn, salt, and dried thyme.
2. Then add the pork belly and boil it for 30 minutes.
3. After this, remove the cooked pork belly from the water and slice.

4. Sprinkle the pork belly with lemon juice.

Nutritional info per serve: Calories 352, Fat 20.4, Fiber 0.2, Carbs 0.5, Protein 35

Ground Pork Pie

Prep time: 15 minutes

Cook time: 25 minutes

Servings:6

Ingredients:

- 1 cup coconut flour
- 3 tablespoons Psyllium husk
- 2 tablespoons butter, softened
- 1 cup ground pork
- 2 oz scallions, chopped
- 1 tablespoon almond flour
- 1 teaspoon chili powder
- 1 teaspoon avocado oil

Method:

1. In the mixing bowl, mix coconut flour, psyllium husk, butter, and almond flour. Knead the dough.
2. After this, put the dough in the baking pan and flatten in the shape of the pie crust with the help of the finger palms.

3. After this, in the mixing bowl, mix ground pork with scallions, chili powder, and avocado oil.
4. Put the mixture over the pie crust and flatten well.
5. Bake the ground pork pie for 25 minutes at 355F.

Nutritional info per serve: Calories 341, Fat 18.8, Fiber 22.8, Carbs 31.1, Protein 18

Lemon Stuffed Pork

Prep time: 10 minutes

Cook time: 30 minutes

Servings: 4

Ingredients:

- 1-pound pork loin
- ½ lemon, sliced
- 1 teaspoon dried rosemary
- ½ teaspoon ground paprika
- 2 tablespoons avocado oil

Method:

1. Slice the pork loin into 4 fillets. Beat the pork fillets with the help of the kitchen hammer.
2. After this, rub the meat with dried rosemary and ground pork.
3. Put the lemon slices on the pork fillets and fold them. Secure the meat with toothpicks and brush with avocado oil.

4. Bake the meat at 360F for 30 minutes. Flip the meat on another side during cooking to avoid burning.

Nutritional info per serve: Calories 288, Fat 16.8, Fiber 0.7, Carbs 1.4, Protein 31.2

Beef and Vegetables Stew

Prep time: 10 minutes

Cook time: 55 minutes

Servings:4

Ingredients:

- 1-pound beef sirloin, chopped
- 1 cup bell pepper, chopped
- 4 cups of water
- 1 tablespoon keto tomato paste
- 1 teaspoon ground coriander
- ½ teaspoon salt
- 1 teaspoon dried sage

Method:

1. Put all ingredients in the saucepan and carefully stir.
2. Bring the mixture to boil, close the lid, and simmer it for 45 minutes on the low heat.

Nutritional info per serve: Calories 224, Fat 7.2, Fiber 0.6, Carbs 3.1, Protein 34.9

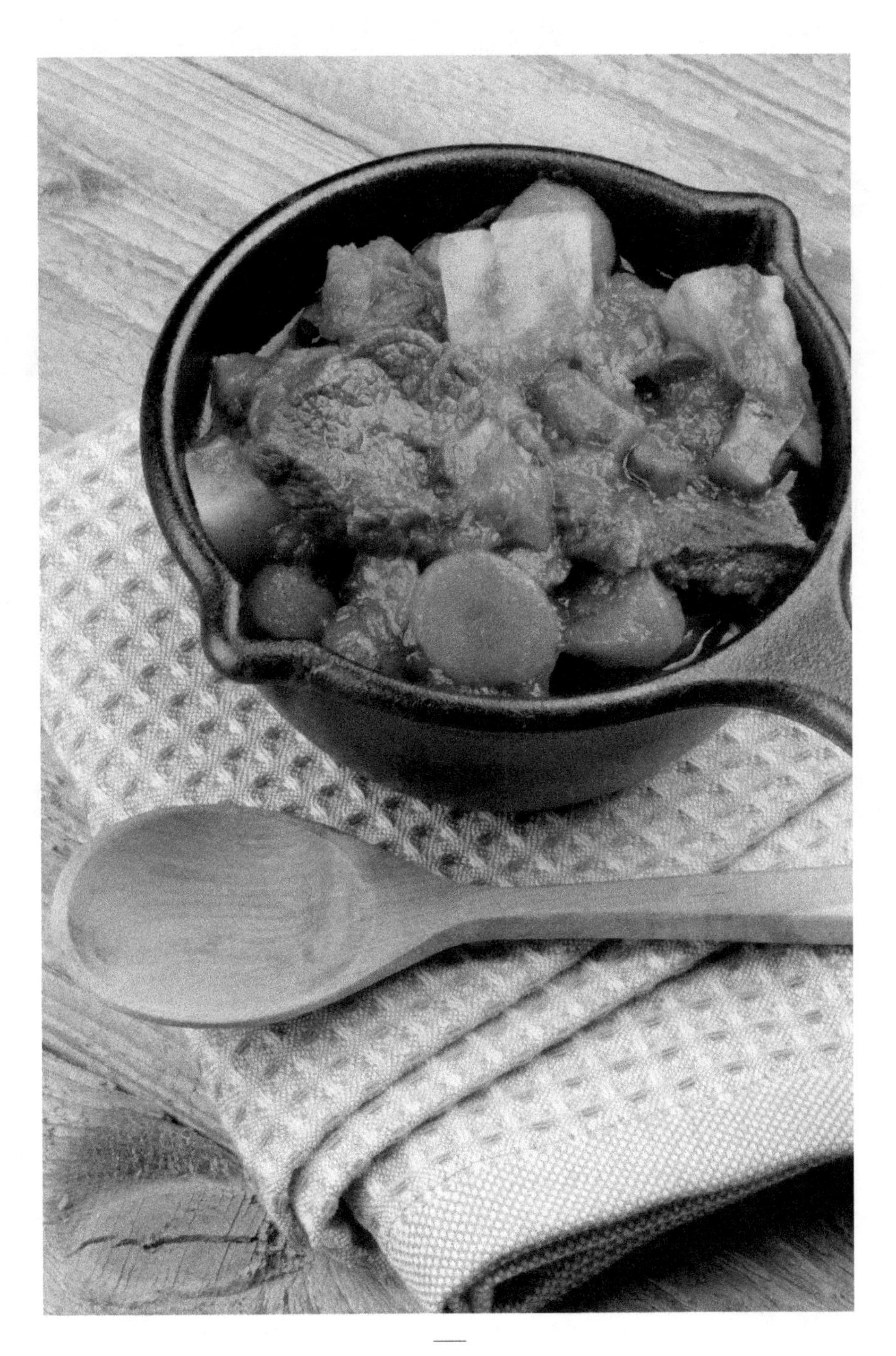

Marinated Pork

Prep time: 25 minutes

Cook time: 20 minutes

Servings: 3

Ingredients:

- 16 oz pork loin, chopped
- ½ cup apple cider vinegar
- 1 tablespoon avocado oil
- 1 teaspoon ground coriander

Method:

1. Mix apple cider vinegar with ground coriander.
2. Put the pork loin in the apple cider vinegar liquid and marinate it for 20 minutes.
3. After this, preheat the skillet well.
4. Add avocado oil and marinated meat.
5. Roast the meat for 20 minutes on the medium heat; stir it from time to time.

Nutritional info per serve: Calories 381, Fat 21.6, Fiber 0.2, Carbs 0.6, Protein 41.4

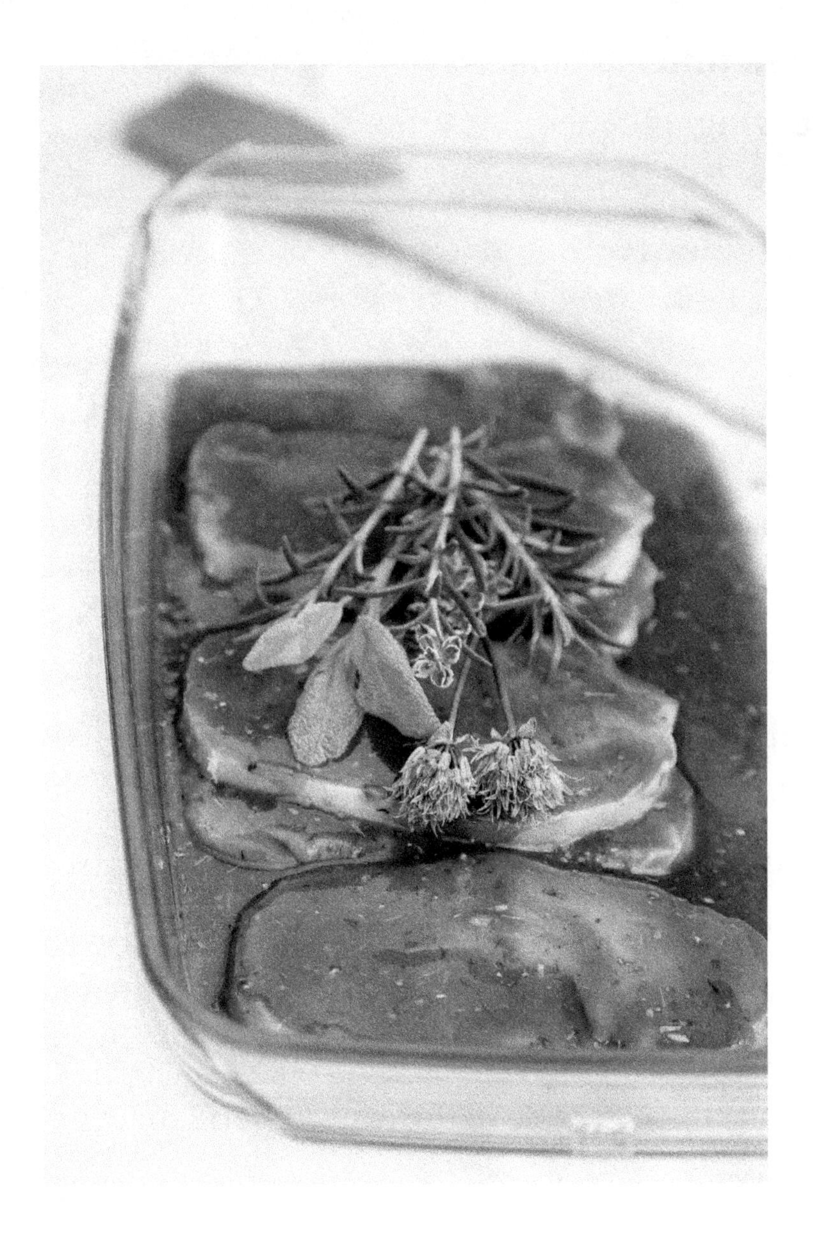

Cheese and Pork Casserole

Prep time: 10 minutes

Cook time: 40 minutes

Servings:5

Ingredients:

- 2 cups ground pork
- 1 cup Cheddar cheese, shredded
- ½ cup coconut cream
- 1 teaspoon dried cilantro
- ½ teaspoon chili powder
- 1 tablespoon butter, softened

Method:

1. Grease the casserole mold with butter.
2. After this, mix ground pork with dried cilantro, coconut cream, and chili powder.
3. Put the mixture in the casserole mold, flatten it in one layer, and top with Cheddar cheese.
4. Bake the casserole in the oven at 360F for 40 minutes.

Nutritional info per serve: Calories 539, Fat 41.6, Fiber 0.6, Carbs 1.8, Protein 38.4

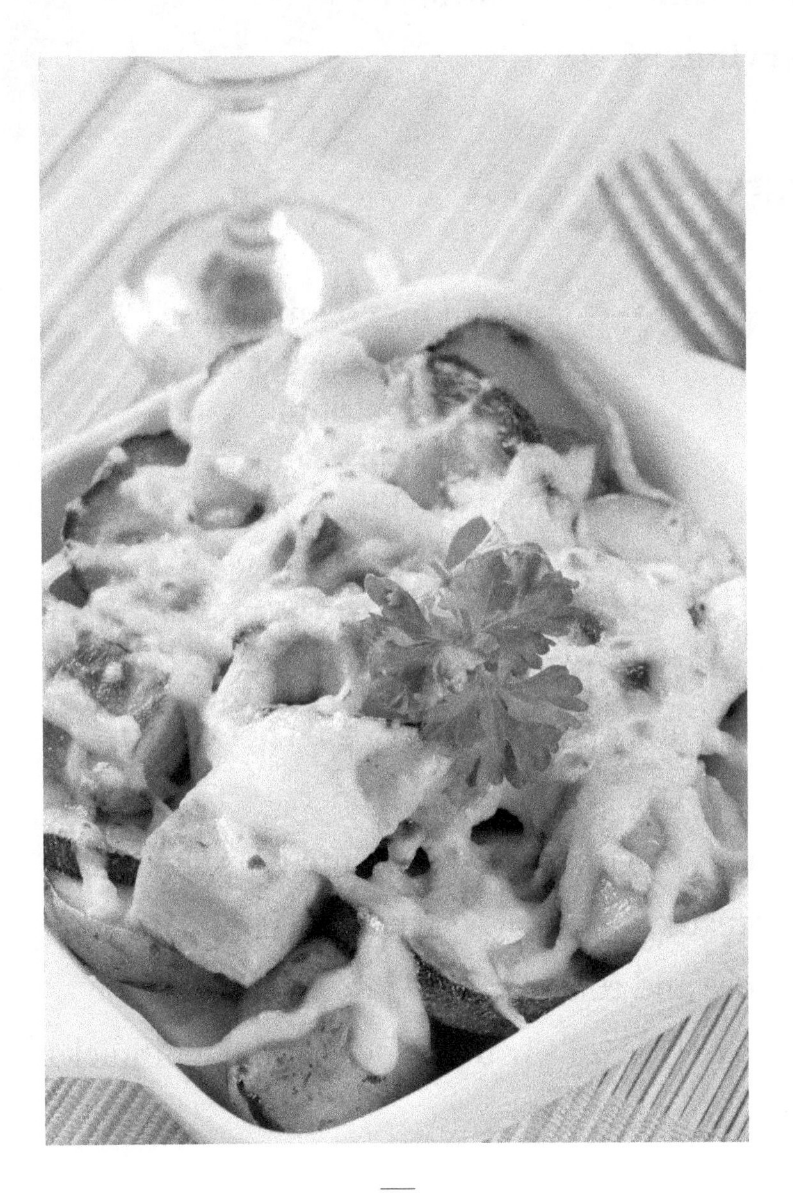

Pork and Cream Cheese Rolls

Prep time: 10 minutes

Cook time: 30 minutes

Servings: 6

Ingredients:

- 3 tablespoons cream cheese
- 2 oz bacon, chopped, cooked
- 1-pound pork sirloin
- 1 teaspoon apple cider vinegar
- 1 teaspoon white pepper
- 1 tablespoon avocado oil

Method:

1. In the mixing bowl, mix cream cheese with chopped bacon and white pepper.
2. Then slice the pork sirloin into 6 servings.
3. Spread every meat serving with cream cheese mixture and roll.
4. Secure the rolls with the help of the toothpicks if needed.

5. Brush the baking pan with avocado oil and put the meat rolls inside.
6. Bake the meat rolls at 360F for 30 minutes.

Nutritional info per serve: Calories 200, Fat 12.7, Fiber 0.2, Carbs 0.6, Protein 19.3

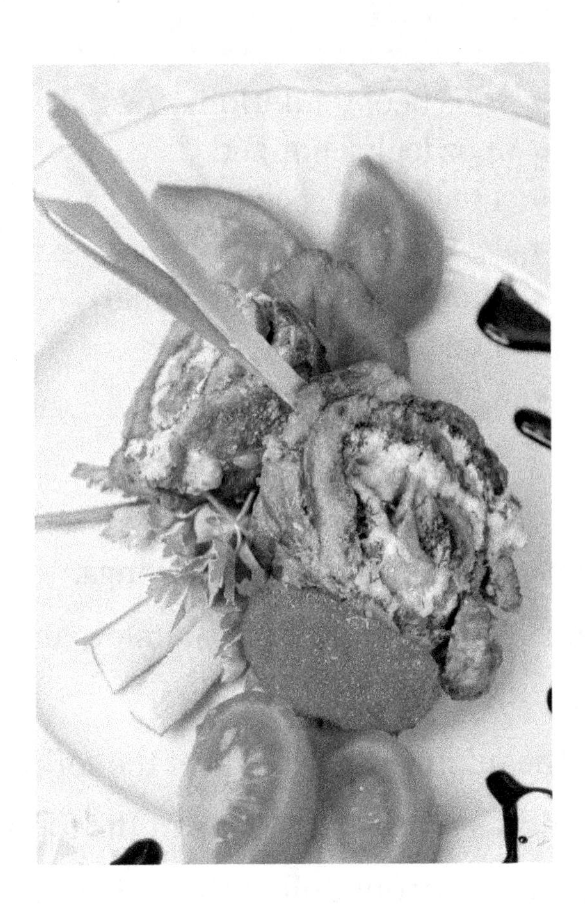

Leek Stuffed Beef

Prep time: 15 minutes

Cook time: 20 minutes

Servings:2

Ingredients:

- 8 oz beef tenderloin
- 4 oz leek, chopped
- 1 teaspoon coconut oil
- ½ teaspoon salt
- 1 tablespoon dried parsley
- 1 oz bacon, chopped
- 1 teaspoon avocado oil

Method:

1. Cut the beef tenderloin into 2 servings.

2. Then mix leek with salt, dried parsley, and chopped bacon.

3. Spread the mixture over the beef tenderloins. Fold the meat and secure with the help of the toothpicks.

4. Then melt the coconut oil in the skillet. Add avocado oil.

5. After this, add beef rolls in the hot oil and roast them for 10 minutes per side on the low heat.

Nutritional info per serve: Calories 368, Fat 19, Fiber 1.2, Carbs 8.5, Protein 39

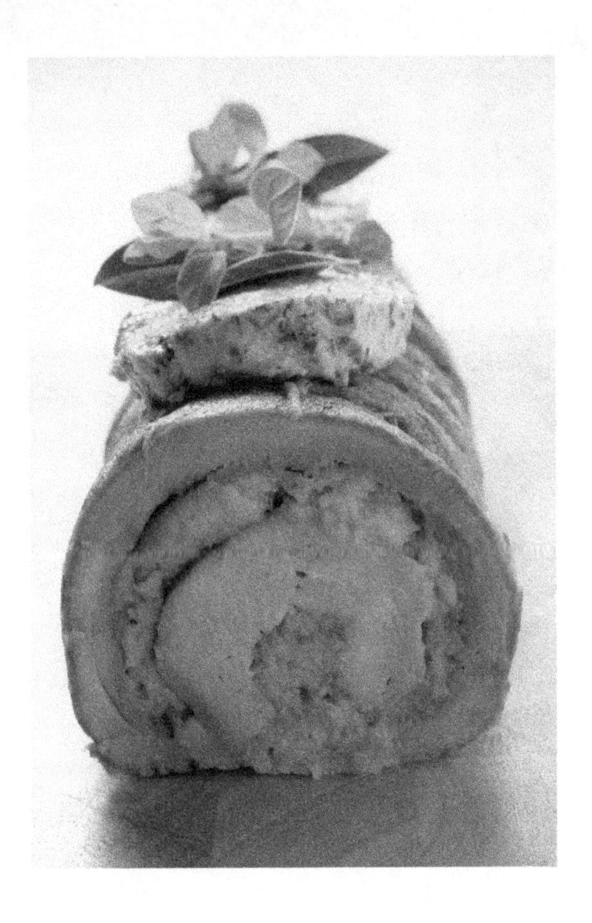

Garlic Pork Loin

Prep time: 10 minutes

Cook time: 50 minutes

Servings: 4

Ingredients:

- 1 teaspoon garlic powder
- 1 garlic clove, diced
- 1-pound pork loin
- 2 tablespoons avocado oil
- ½ teaspoon salt

Method:

1. Rub the pork loin with salt, diced garlic, and garlic powder.
2. Then sprinkle the meat with avocado oil and wrap in the foil.
3. Bake the pork loin in the preheated to 360F oven for 50 minutes.

Nutritional info per serve: Calories 340, Fat 22.8, Fiber 0.1, Carbs 0.8, Protein 31.2

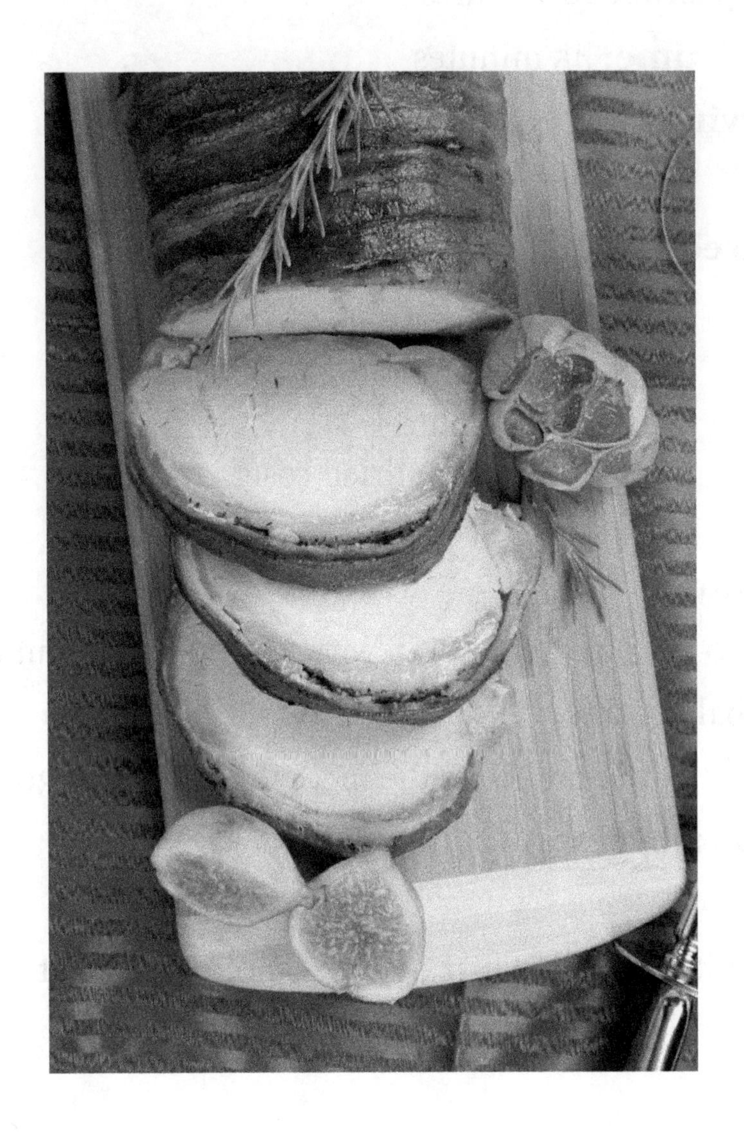

Butter Pork

Prep time: 10 minutes

Cook time: 45 minutes

Servings:4

Ingredients:

- 1-pound pork tenderloin
- ¼ cup butter
- 1 teaspoon dried rosemary

Method:

1. Rub the pork tenderloin with rosemary and put in the baking tray.
2. Add butter and bake the meat in the oven at 360F for 45 minutes.

Nutritional info per serve: Calories 265, Fat 15.5, Fiber 0.1, Carbs 0.2, Protein 29.8

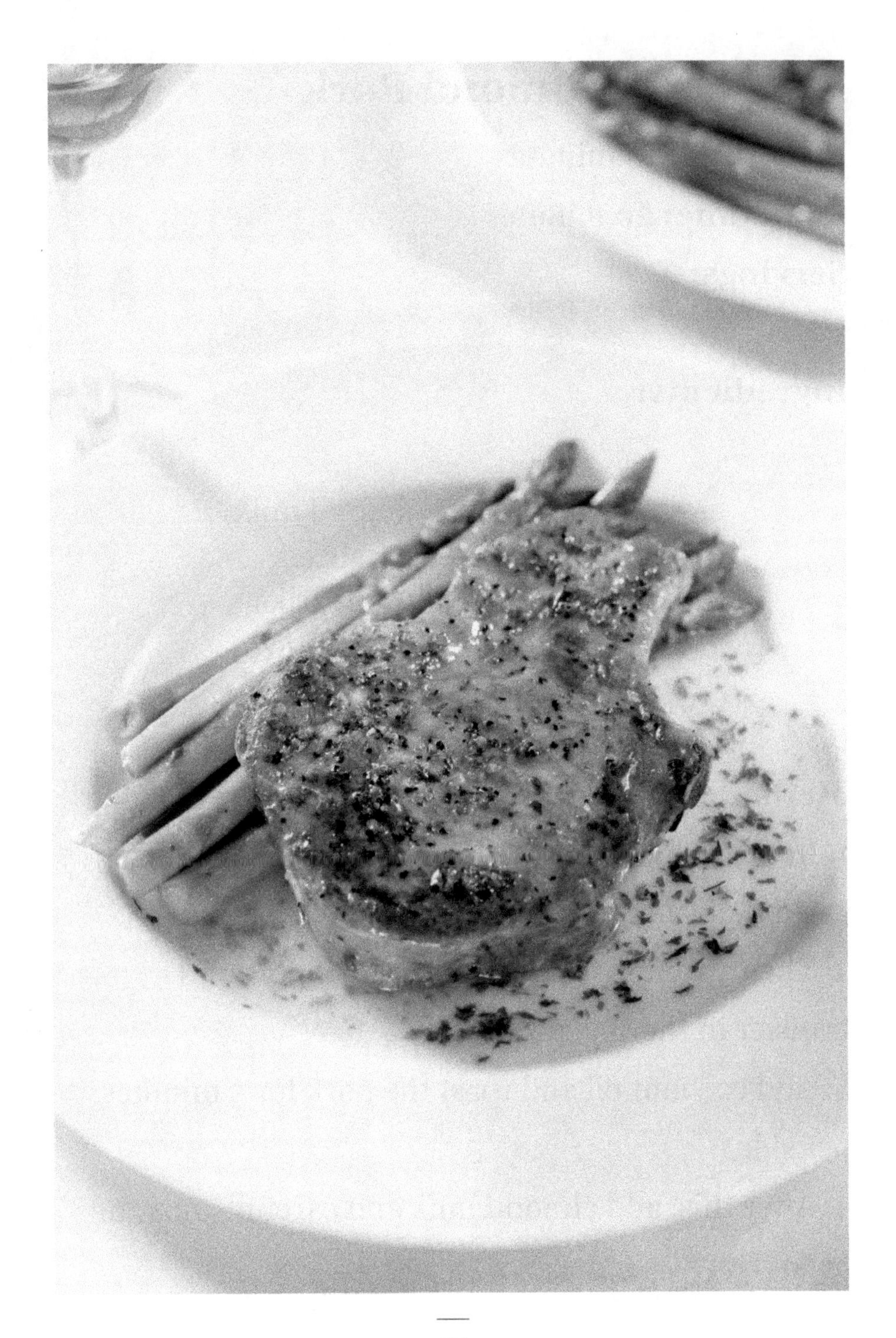

Almond Pork

Prep time: 10 minutes

Cook time: 20 minutes

Servings: 4

Ingredients:

- ½ cup organic almond milk
- 1-pound pork loin, sliced
- 1 teaspoon ground paprika
- 1 teaspoon ground nutmeg
- 1 tablespoon coconut oil

Method:

1. In the shallow bowl, mix ground paprika and ground nutmeg.
2. Then sprinkle the pork loin with spices and transfer in the skillet.
3. Add coconut oil and roast the pork for 5 minutes per side.
4. After this, add almond milk and carefully mix the meat.

5. Close the lid and cook the pork on medium-low heat for 10 minutes.

Nutritional info per serve: Calories 377, Fat 26.6, Fiber 1, Carbs 2.2, Protein 31.8

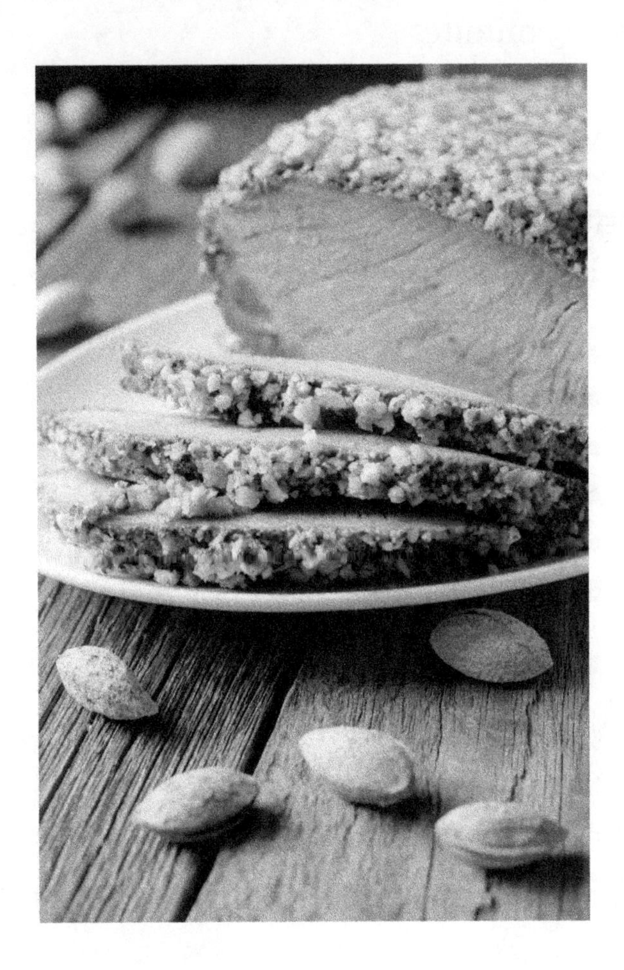

Ketogenic Dessert Recipes

Butter Truffles

Prep time: 10 minutes

Cook time: 5 minutes

Servings: 10

Ingredients:

- 3 oz dark chocolate, chopped
- 2 tablespoons butter
- ⅔ cup coconut cream
- 2 tablespoons Erythritol
- ¼ teaspoon vanilla extract
- 1 teaspoon of cocoa powder

Method:

1. Melt the chocolate and mix it with butter.

2. Add coconut cream, Erythritol, and vanilla extract.

3. Then make the small balls (truffles) and coat them in the cocoa powder.

4. Refrigerate the dessert for 10-15 minutes before serving.

Nutritional info per serve: Calories 103, Fat 8.7, Fiber 0.7, Carbs 6.1, Protein 1.1

Pecan Brownies

Prep time: 15 minutes

Cook time: 25 minutes

Servings:4

Ingredients:

- 3 eggs, beaten
- 2 tablespoons cocoa powder
- 2 teaspoons Erythritol
- ½ cup coconut flour
- 2 pecans, chopped
- ½ cup of coconut milk

Method:

1. In the mixing bowl, mix eggs with cocoa powder, Erythritol, coconut flour, pecans, and coconut milk.
2. Stir the mixture until smooth and pour it in the brownie mold. Flatten the surface of the brownie batter if needed.
3. Bake it at 360F for 25 minutes.
4. When the brownie is cooked, cut it into bars.

Nutritional info per serve: Calories 178, Fat 16, Fiber 2.8, Carbs 5.4, Protein 6.3

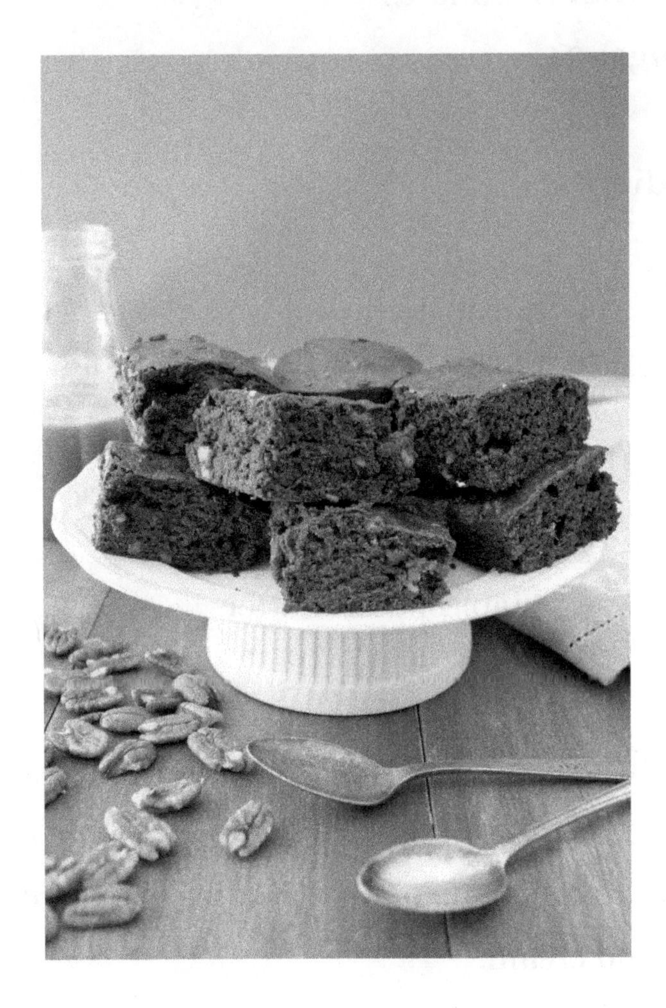

Flaxseeds Doughnuts

Prep time: 20 minutes

Cook time: 12 minutes

Servings: 24

Ingredients:

- ¼ cup erythritol
- ¼ cup flaxseed meal
- ¾ cup coconut flour
- 1 teaspoon baking powder
- 1 teaspoon vanilla extract
- 2 eggs, beaten
- 3 tablespoons butter
- ¼ cup heavy cream

Method:

1. In the mixing bowl, mix erythritol, flaxseed meal, coconut flour, baking powder, vanilla extract, eggs, butter, and cream.
2. Knead the soft dough and roll up it.

3. Cut the dough into doughnuts with the help of the cutter and put in the lined with a baking paper baking tray.
4. Bake the doughnuts in the preheated to 365F oven for 12 minutes or until the dessert is light brown.

Nutritional info per serve: Calories 44, Fat 3, Fiber 1.8, Carbs 3, Protein 1.2

Jelly Bears

Prep time: 20 minutes

Cook time: 10 minutes

Servings:7

Ingredients:

- 1 cup of water
- 2 oz strawberries, mashed
- 1 tablespoon gelatin
- 1 teaspoon Erythritol

Method:

1. Mix water with mashed strawberries and Erythritol.
2. Bring the liquid to boil and chill for 10 minutes.
3. Then add gelatin and stir the liquid until it is smooth.
4. Pour it in the silicon molds with the shape of bears and refrigerate until solid.

Nutritional info per serve: Calories 6, Fat 0, Fiber 0.6, Carbs 0.6, Protein 0.9

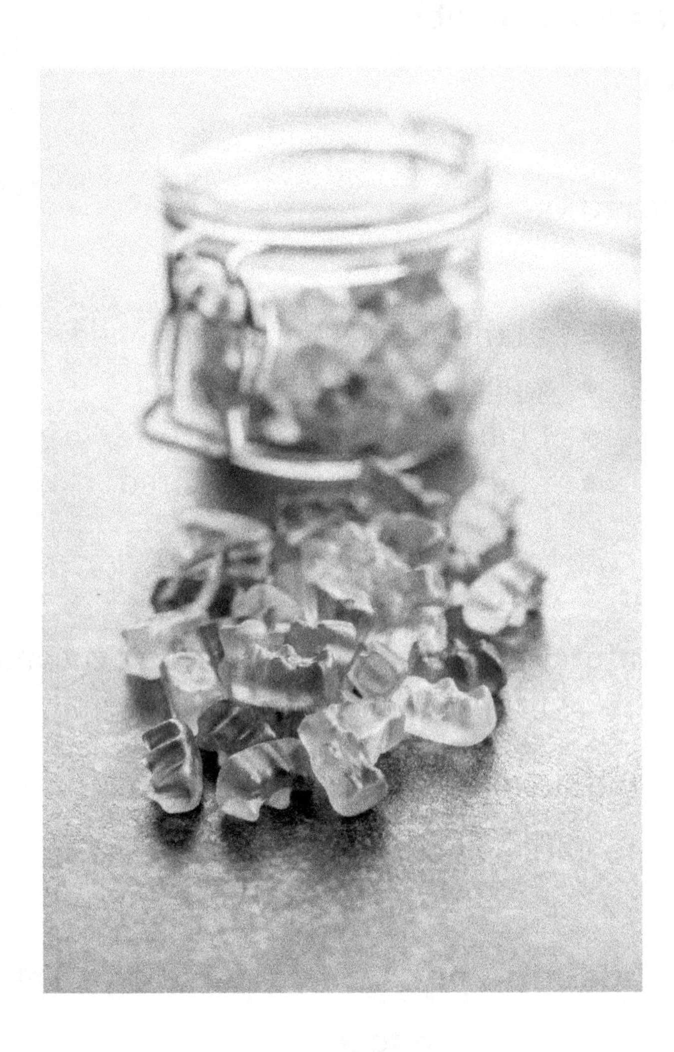

Pecan Candies

Prep time: 10 minutes

Cook time: 0 minutes

Servings: 6

Ingredients:

- 5 tablespoons butter, softened
- 4 pecans, chopped
- 1 tablespoon Erythritol
- 1 tablespoon coconut shred

Method:

1. Mix butter with pecans, Erythritol, and coconut shred.
2. Make the small balls from the pecan mixture and refrigerate until solid.

Nutritional info per serve: Calories 155, Fat 16.8, Fiber 1.1, Carbs 1.6, Protein 1.2

Cocoa Pie

Prep time: 10 minutes

Cook time: 40 minutes

Servings:5

Ingredients:

- 1 teaspoon baking powder
- 1 teaspoon vanilla extract
- 2 eggs, beaten
- 4 tablespoons cocoa powder
- 2 tablespoons swerve
- 8 tablespoons coconut cream
- 4 teaspoon coconut flour
- 1 teaspoon avocado oil

Method:

1. In the mixing bowl, mix baking powder with vanilla extract, eggs, cocoa powder, swerve, coconut cream, and coconut flour.
2. Stir the mixture until you get a smooth batter.
3. Then brush the baking pan with avocado oil and pour the pie batter inside.

4. Bake the pie at 360F for 40 minutes.

Nutritional info per serve: Calories 105, Fat 8.4, Fiber 2.6, Carbs 6.3, Protein 3.8

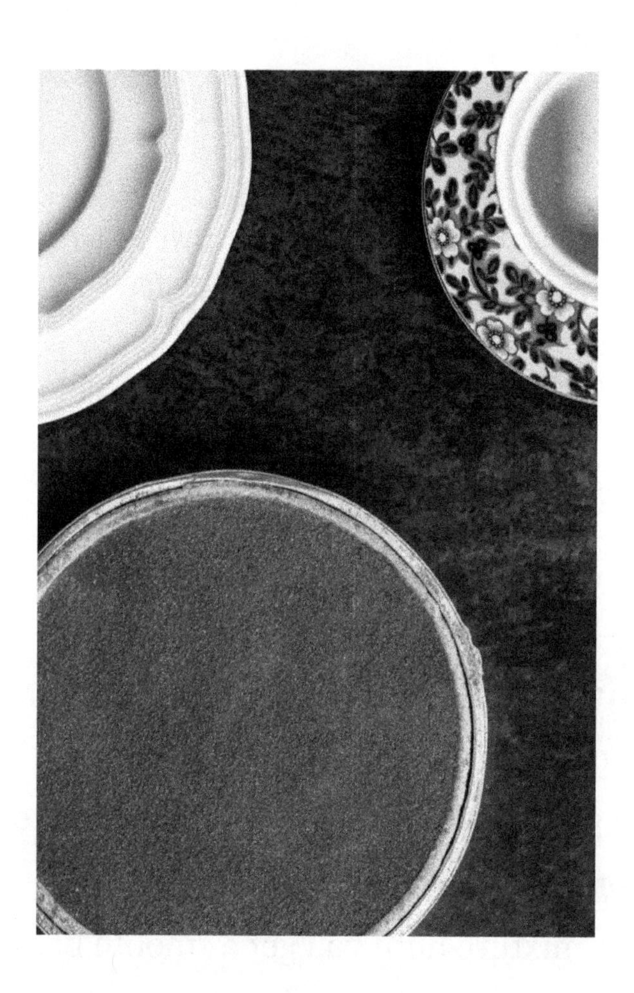

Cream Jelly

Prep time: 2 hours

Cook time: 1 minute

Servings: 5

Ingredients:

- 2 tablespoons Erythritol
- 1 teaspoon vanilla extract
- 2 cups heavy cream
- 2 tablespoons gelatin

Method:

1. Mix gelatin with ¼ cup of cream and microwave for 1 minute.
2. Then mix gelatin mixture with remaining heavy cream, vanilla extract, and Erythritol. Stir the liquid carefully.
3. Pour it in the silicone molds and refrigerate.
4. When the jelly is solid, the dessert is cooked.

Nutritional info per serve: Calories 177, Fat 17.8, Fiber 0, Carbs 1.5, Protein 3.4

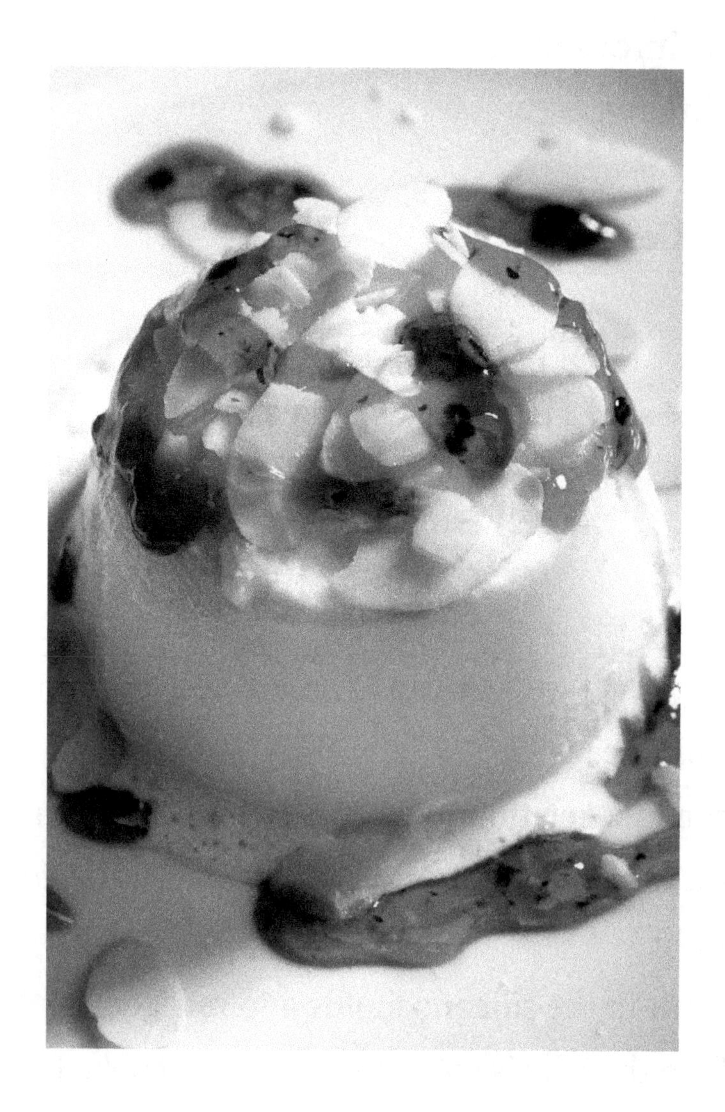

Vanilla Mousse

Prep time: 7 minutes

Cook time: 7 minutes

Servings:3

Ingredients:

- 2 blackberries, halved
- 1 cup heavy cream
- ½ teaspoon vanilla extract
- 2 teaspoon swerve
- 4 tablespoons butter

Method:

1. Whip the heavy cream and mix it with butter, swerve, and vanilla extract.
2. Whisk the mousse until homogenous.
3. Then transfer it in the serving cups and top with blackberries.

Nutritional info per serve: Calories 276, Fat 30.2, Fiber 0, Carbs 1.4, Protein 1

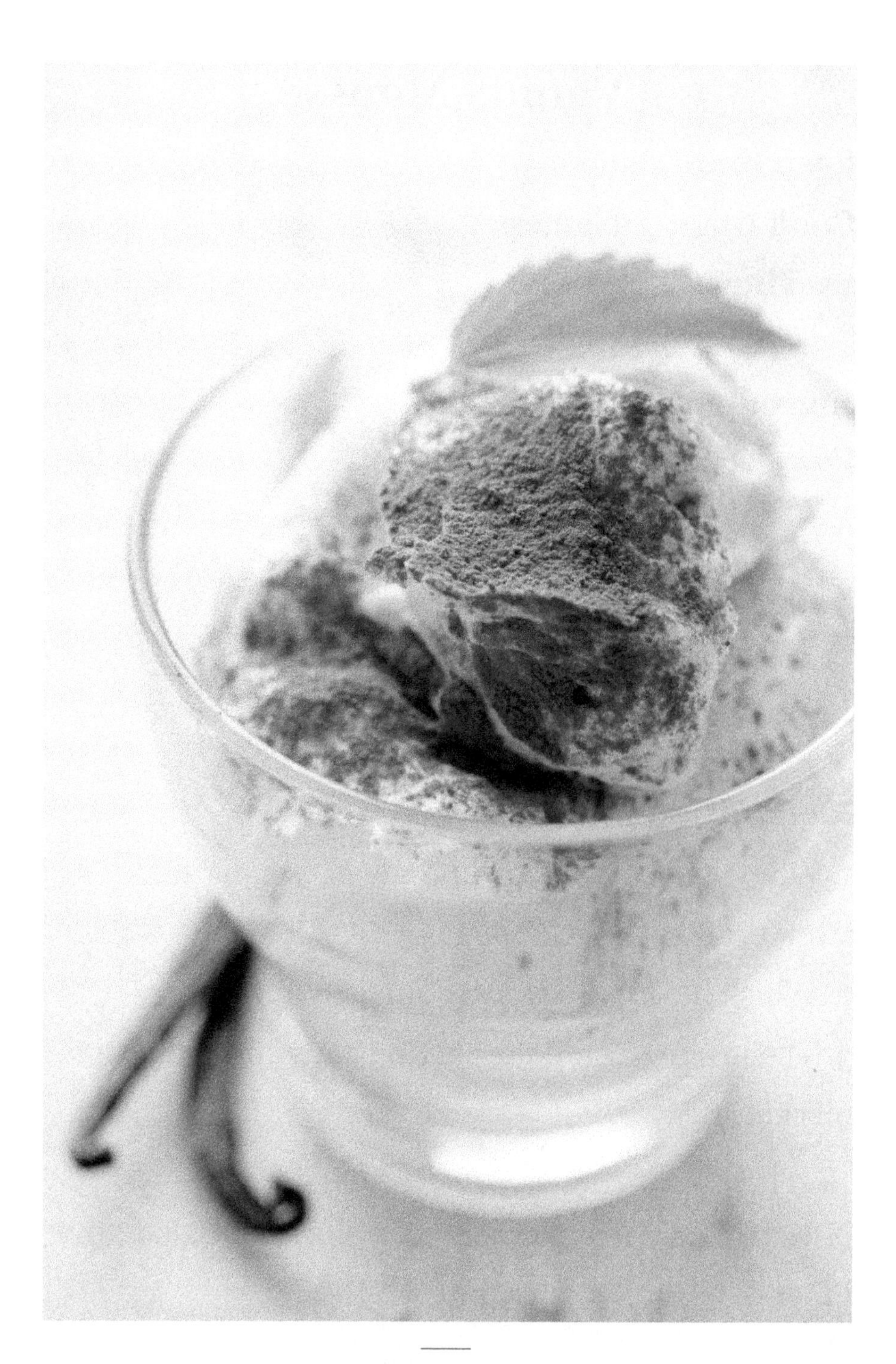

Cheese Pie

Prep time: 10 minutes

Cook time: 40 minutes

Servings: 12

Ingredients:

- 1 cup coconut, shredded
- 2 tablespoons flax seeds
- ¼ cup of coconut oil
- ½ cup heavy cream
- 1 cup cream cheese
- 3 tablespoons Erythritol
- 1 teaspoon vanilla extract
- 1 tablespoon gelatin

Method:

1. Mix the shredded coconut with flax seeds, coconut oil, heavy cream, cream cheese, Erythritol, and vanilla extract.
2. Whisk the mixture until smooth and add gelatin.
3. Start to preheat the liquid until gelatin is melted.

4. Then transfer the pie in the baking mold and refrigerate for 40 minutes.

Nutritional info per serve: Calories 157, Fat 15.7, Fiber 0.9, Carbs 2, Protein 2.5

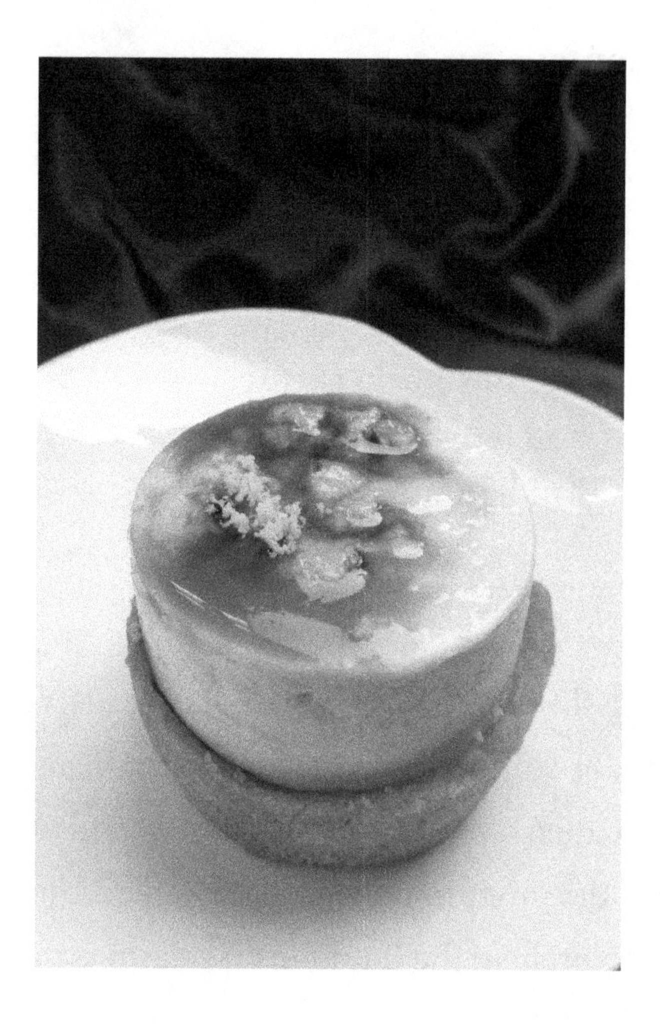

Avocado Mousse

Prep time: 15 minutes

Cook time: 0 minutes

Servings:4

Ingredients:

- 1 avocado, peeled, pitted, chopped
- 1/3 cup coconut cream
- 1 tablespoon Erythritol
- 1 teaspoon vanilla extract

Method:

1. Blend the avocado until smooth.
2. Then add coconut cream, Erythritol, and vanilla extract.
3. Carefully stir the cooked mousse and transfer it in the serving bowl.

Nutritional info per serve: Calories 152, Fat 14.6, Fiber 3.8, Carbs 5.6, Protein 1.4

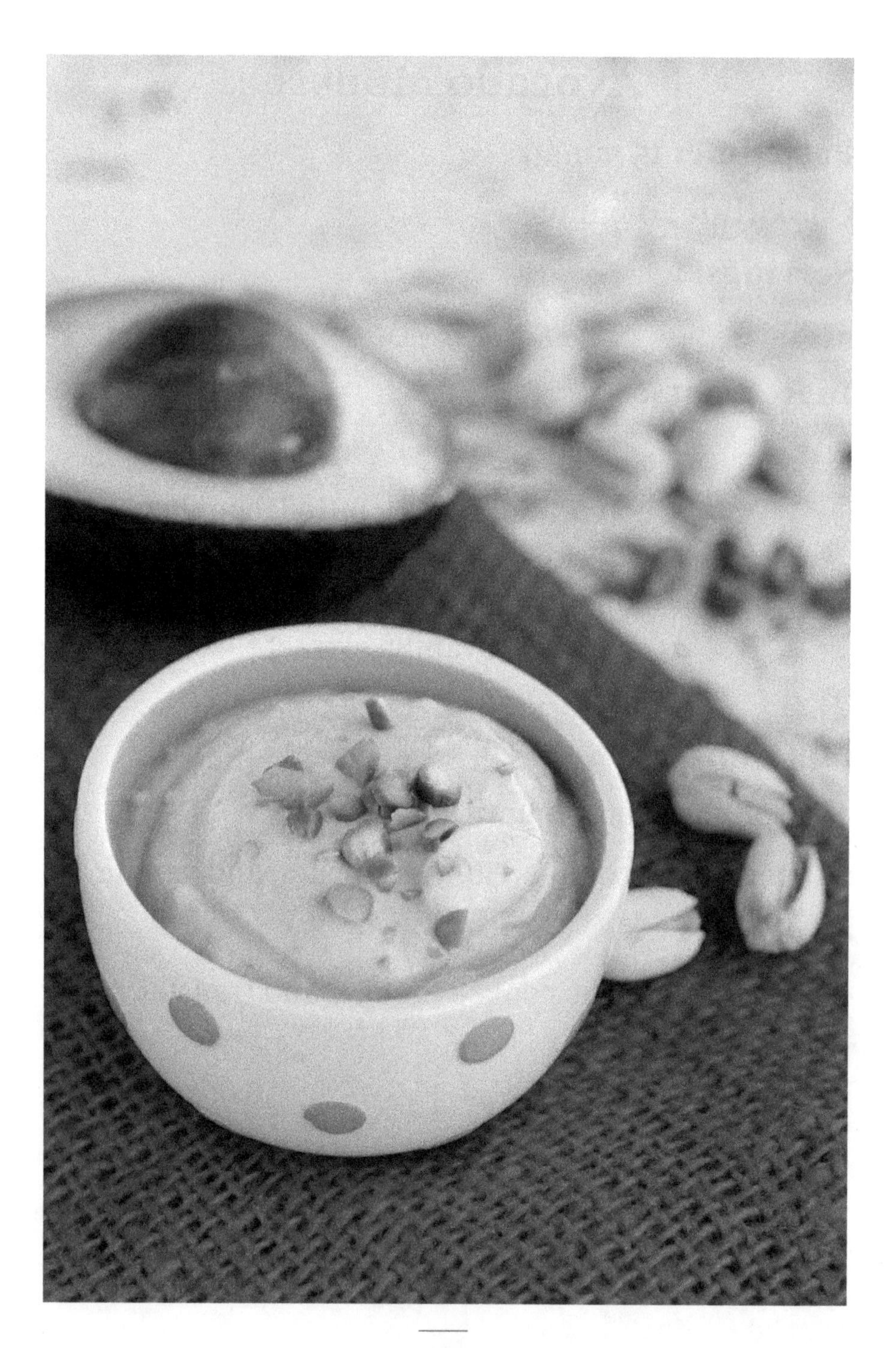

Chocolate Pie

Prep time: 10 minutes

Cook time: 30 minutes

Servings: 8

Ingredients:

- 3 tablespoons butter, softened
- ½ cup heavy cream
- 1 teaspoon baking powder
- 1 cup coconut flour
- 1 oz dark chocolate, chopped

Method:

1. Mix butter with baking powder, coconut flour, and heavy cream.
2. Then transfer the mixture in the non-stick baking pan. Flatten the surface of the pie with the help of the spatula and top with chopped chocolate.
3. Bake the pie at 360F for 30 minutes.

Nutritional info per serve: Calories 91, Fat 8.4, Fiber 0.8, Carbs 3.6, Protein 0.7

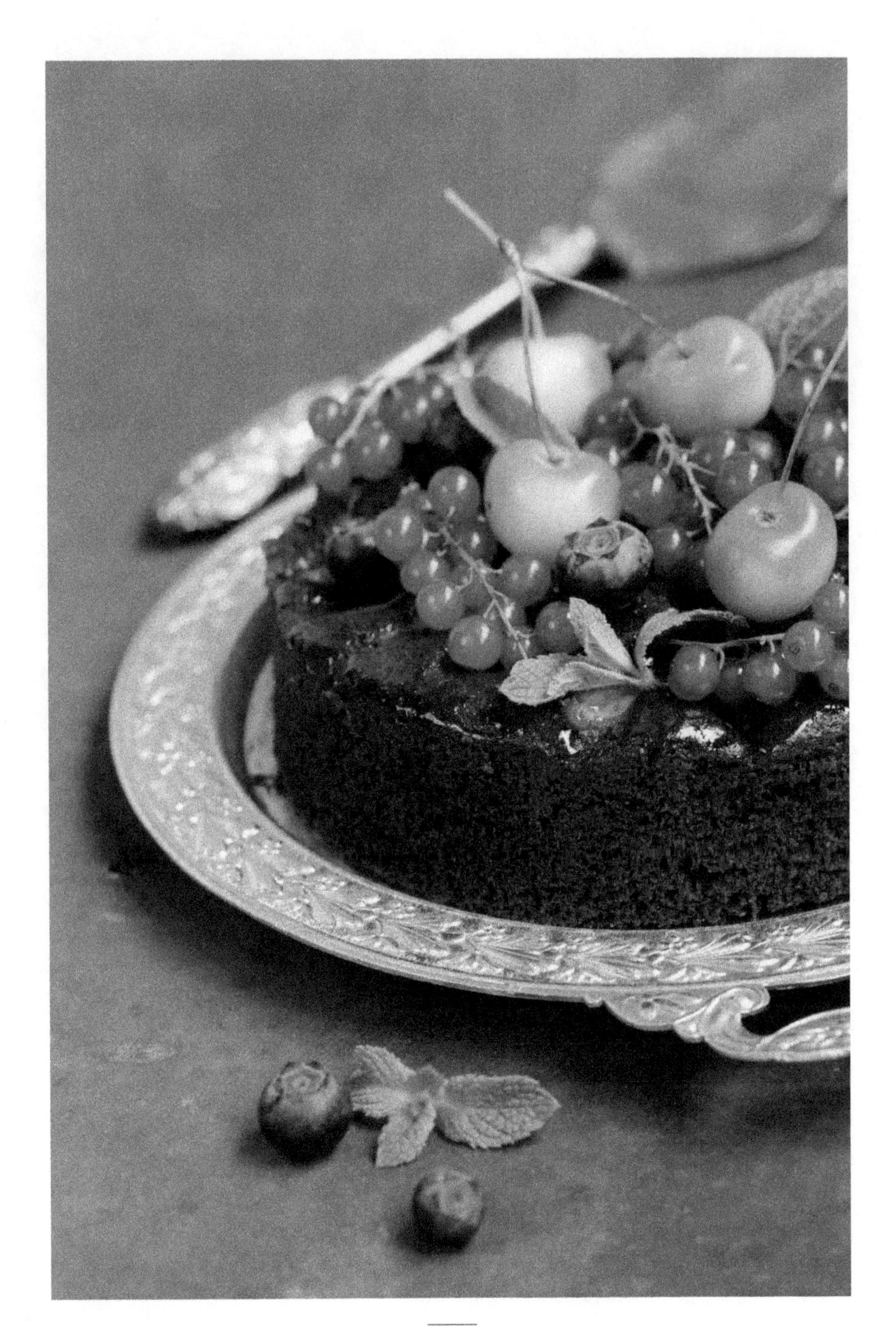

CPSIA information can be obtained
at www.ICGtesting.com
Printed in the USA
BVHW091051240221
600902BV00004B/1145